See what people are saying about
The Hungry Girl Diet . . .

After four weeks on the plan:

"I'm ecstatic with my weight loss. I had been on a plateau [using another diet plan], and this diet gave me the boost I needed to get back on track. **Simple, effective, and fabulous."** —Michelle M. (LOST 16 POUNDS)

"LOVE IT! Thank you for developing it for people like me. I enjoy food. . . . I'm glad there is a plan out there that I can use and not feel like I'm missing out on everything." —Stevenie E. (LOST 11 POUNDS)

"I found something that works for me, and I enjoy eating all that food!!! The food was healthy, but also delicious. **I feel like I have learned how to eat better."** —Mary G. (LOST 16 POUNDS)

"I never felt hungry on the plan, which makes it stand out from others. I always felt hungry or unsatisfied when I was [on other diets], but I felt like I was always eating on this plan." —Erin L. (LOST 12 POUNDS)

Continued success with the plan:

"I could not for the life of me get those last 40 pounds off without the help of your book! **I now have a tool book of everything I need to stay on track *for life*."** —Robin C. (LOST 40 POUNDS)

"It's so amazing to eat big portions of real food (using recipes that even I can prepare!) **and still lose weight."** —Colleen M. (LOST 30 POUNDS)

"I feel great and have so much more energy. **The HG Diet helped me reach my goal weight for my wedding—I felt so beautiful."** —Katherine R. (LOST 37 POUNDS)

"I have lost weight with diet pills and other diets only to gain it back. This diet is easy to stay on—I will continue until I reach my goal. **I have found a new lease on life."** —Tammy T. (LOST 30 POUNDS)

"Keeping my husband satisfied on this plan has been easy! The Hungry Girl Diet lays everything at your feet: **effective tips, cheerful encouragement, diverse menus,** and fast simple recipes." —Penny K. (LOST 40 POUNDS) and Mitch K. (LOST 48 POUNDS)

"I love how easy it is to follow and how tasty the food is. **The diet works,** even for people who are always busy." —Stephanie M. (LOST 81 POUNDS)

"We love the recipes because they are **delicious, flavorful, and filling!** We have never felt like we were on a diet and were always satisfied!" —Valerie M. (LOST 91 POUNDS) and Ron M. (LOST 40 POUNDS)

Also by Lisa Lillien

Hungry Girl:
Recipes and Survival Strategies for Guilt-Free Eating in the Real World

Hungry Girl 200 Under 200:
200 Recipes Under 200 Calories

Hungry Girl 1-2-3:
The Easiest, Most Delicious, Guilt-Free Recipes on the Planet

Hungry Girl Happy Hour:
75 Recipes for Amazingly Fantastic Guilt-Free Cocktails & Party Foods

Hungry Girl 300 Under 300:
300 Breakfast, Lunch & Dinner Dishes Under 300 Calories

Hungry Girl Supermarket Survival:
Aisle by Aisle, HG-Style!

HUNGRY GIRL TO THE MAX!
The Ultimate Guilt-Free Cookbook

Hungry Girl 200 Under 200 Just Desserts:
200 Recipes Under 200 Calories

The Hungry Girl Diet

Hungry Girl:
The Official Survival Guides: Tips & Tricks for Guilt-Free Eating
(audio book)

Hungry Girl Chew the Right Thing:
Supreme Makeovers for 50 Foods You Crave
(recipe cards)

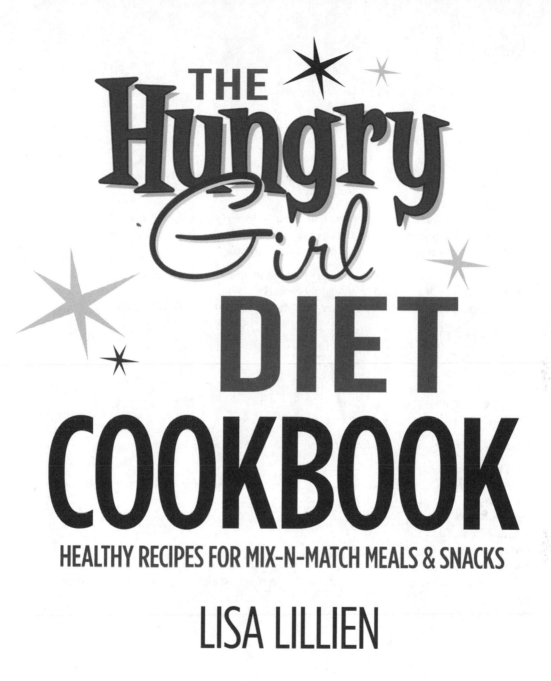

THE Hungry Girl DIET COOKBOOK

HEALTHY RECIPES FOR MIX-N-MATCH MEALS & SNACKS

LISA LILLIEN

St. Martin's Griffin 🅜 New York

THE HUNGRY GIRL DIET COOKBOOK: HEALTHY RECIPES FOR MIX-N-MATCH MEALS & SNACKS. Copyright © 2015 by Hungry Girl, Inc. All rights reserved. Printed in the United States of America. For information, address St. Martin's Press, 175 Fifth Avenue, New York, N.Y. 10010.

www.stmartins.com

Cover design by Ralph Fowler and Julie Leonard
Book design by Ralph Fowler
Illustrations by Jack Pullan
Food styling by Cindie Flannigan
Photography by Heather Winters

The Library of Congress has cataloged the hardcover edition as follows:

Lillien, Lisa.
    The hungry girl diet cookbook : healthy recipes for mix-n-match meals & snacks / Lisa Lillien. — First edition.
        p. cm.
    Includes index.
    ISBN 978-1-250-06884-2 (hardcover)
    ISBN 978-1-4668-8151-8 (e-book)
    1. Reducing diets—Recipes.   2. Nutrition.   3. Women—Health and hygiene.   4. Cookbooks.
I. Title.
    RM222.2.L47773 2015
    641.5'635—dc23

                                                                                2015007354

ISBN 978-1-250-08041-7 (trade paperback)

Our books may be purchased in bulk for promotional, educational, or business use. Please contact your local bookseller or the Macmillan Corporate and Premium Sales Department at (800) 221-7945, extension 5442, or by e-mail at MacmillanSpecialMarkets@macmillan.com.

First St. Martin's Griffin Trade Paperback Edition: December 2015

10 9 8 7 6 5 4 3 2 1

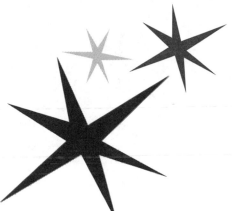

This book is dedicated to all the loyal Hungry Girl fans and daily-email subscribers who more or less *demanded* a Hungry Girl Diet and this subsequent cookbook! THANK YOU. You are the inspiration for all things Hungry Girl and are so appreciated.

CONTENTS

Ch 2: Growing Oatmeal, Oat Bran, Quinoa & More

Ch 3: Protein-Packed Fruit Bowls & Breakfast Smoothies

Ch 4: Pumped-Up Pancakes, French Toast & Crepes

LUNCHES & DINNERS

Ch 5: Stir-Frys, Skillets & Grills

Ch 6: Tacos, Tostadas, and More

Ch 7: Soups, Stews & Bowls

Ch 8: Salads

Ch 9: Sandwiches, Burgers & Wraps

Ch 10: Lettuce Wraps & Lettuce Cups

Ch 11: Pasta & Pasta Swaps

Ch 12: Foil Packs & HG Bakes

SNACKS

Ch 13: Crispy, Crunchy

GO-TO GUIDE FOR GROCERY SHOPPING, MONEY SAVING, MEAL PREPPING & MORE

Acknowledgments

Jamie Goldberg—thank you so much for putting your heart and soul into this book, for your unparalleled work ethic, and for your continued passion for all things Hungry Girl. Looking forward to the next decade of calorie slashing and beyond!

Tremendous thank-yous go out to the following members of the talented and tireless HG team. From recipe testing to nutritional number crunching, this book wouldn't exist without your help!

Lynn Bettencourt
Dana DeRuyck
Callie Pegadiotes
Michelle Ferrand
Amanda Pisani
Erin Norcross
Julie Leonard
Katie Killeavy

I'd also like to thank the rest of the incredibly hardworking Hungry Girl staff . . .

Alison Kreuch
Sue Williams
Gina Muscato
Lisa Mittin
Nick Souza

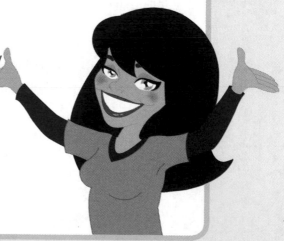

. . . and extended Hungry Girl family!

Neeti Madan

Jennifer Enderlin

John Karle

Anne Marie Tallberg

Elizabeth Catalano

James Sinclair

Cheryl Mamaril

Jeanne-Marie Hudson

Stephanie Davis

Tracey Guest

John Vaccaro

Bill Stankey

Tom Fineman

Jeff Becker

Jackie Mgido

Jennifer Fleming

Olga Gatica

Heather Winters

Cindie Flannigan

Jack Pullan

Ralph Fowler

David Grotto, MS, RDN, LDN

Elizabeth Hodson

Last but not least, all my love and gratitude go out to my amazing parents and siblings, my lovable and supportive husband, and my furry children . . .

Florence and Maurice Lillien

Meri Lillien

Jay Lillien

Daniel Schneider

Lolly and Jackson

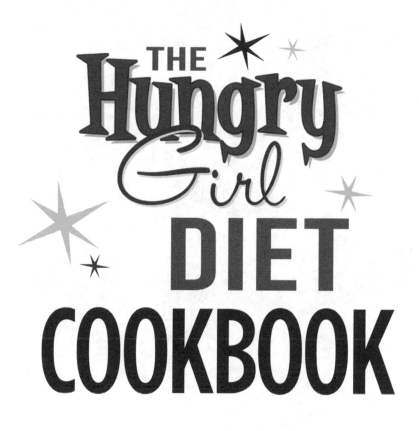

THE

Hungry
Girl
DIET
COOKBOOK

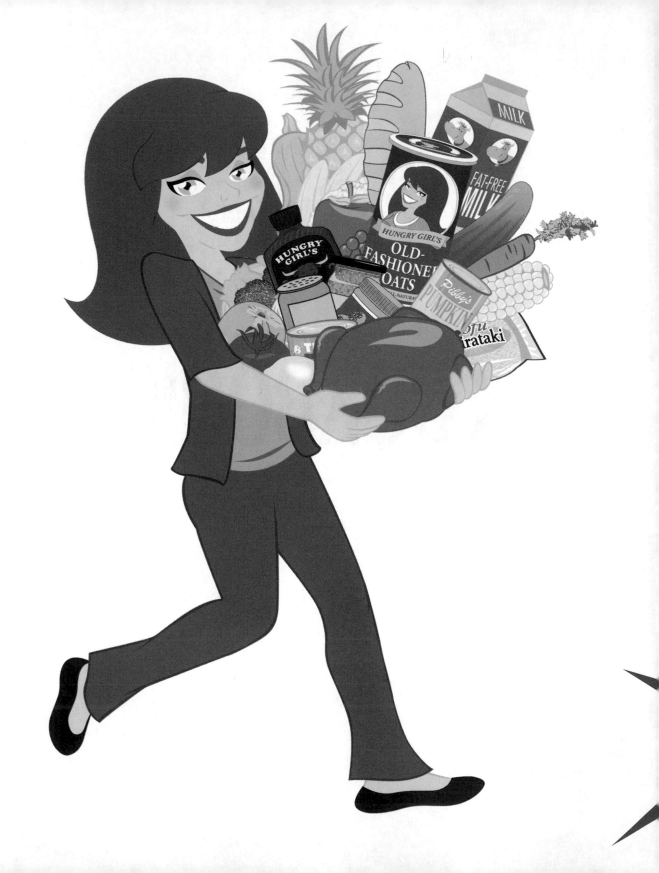

INTRODUCTION

Welcome to
The Hungry Girl Diet Cookbook!

In this follow-up to the #1 *New York Times* Best Seller *The Hungry Girl Diet,* you'll find 200 easy and amazing new recipes for breakfasts, lunch & dinner dishes, and snacks—all of which fit perfectly into the Hungry Girl Diet plan! Whether or not you're following the HG diet, you'll LOVE these Hungry Girl creations. They're simple, delicious, satisfying, and nutritious . . .

Dig in!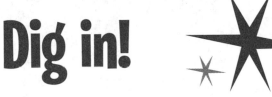

FAQs

Got questions? We've got answers . . .

What is the Hungry Girl Diet?

After 10 years of guilt-free recipes, foods finds, tips 'n tricks, and more, the Hungry Girl fans more or less demanded a *specific* weight-loss plan that combines everything they know and love about HG. The resulting dietitian-approved plan has helped countless women and men achieve their weight-loss goals. Flexible yet foolproof, it emphasizes lean protein, fresh fruits and veggies, large portions, and craving-busting swaps! Each day consists of three meals and three snacks, totaling about 1,300 calories. There's also a 1,500-calorie option. Flip to page 7 for an at-a-glance guide, and get more info about the diet at hungry-girl.com/diet . . . and in the pages of *The Hungry Girl Diet*!

Why a Hungry Girl Diet cookbook?

Among other things, *The Hungry Girl Diet* features a four-week jump-start plan, one that can be repeated as often as needed until reaching your goal weight. And we were THRILLED to hear from masses of dieters who did just that! While the diet book features 60 or so customizable recipes, it became clear that Hungry Girl dieters were HUNGRY FOR MORE. And so, *The Hungry Girl Diet Cookbook* was born . . .

Do I NEED the diet book to use this book?

Technically, no. Each day on the Hungry Girl Diet consists of three HG-Diet meals and three HG-Diet snacks. So you could mix and match these recipes to your heart's content, and you'd be well on your way to weight loss. In fact, the recipes in this cookbook can be enjoyed as a part of any flexible weight-loss or weight-management plan.

However . . . *The Hungry Girl Diet* is more than just meals and snacks. While virtually all the recipes in this book are quick and easy, the diet book has some *super-simple* staple meals that are more like food assembly than full-on recipes . . . plus a large list of grab-n-go snacks. If you're going to follow the plan for a while, you'll want these non-recipe, plan-approved options!

The Hungry Girl Diet also includes a comprehensive guide to dining out on the plan, secrets to success, invaluable tips for avoiding common diet missteps, a massive section on maintenance, and so much more. For the fastest and most effective weight loss (that stays lost!), you'll definitely want a copy of *The Hungry Girl Diet*.

How do I incorporate these recipes into the Hungry Girl Diet?

If you want to get a structured start, begin by following the four-week diet plan laid out in *The Hungry Girl Diet*—with specific meal 'n snack guidance, it was thoughtfully developed to kick off your weight loss in a *major* way.

Ready to dive in right here and now? Just flip to page 7 for A Day on the Hungry Girl Diet. Then mix and match your perfect meal plan, changing it up day by day!

And any time you need a little more structure, just return to the four-week plan . . .

What makes these recipes different from the ones in other Hungry Girl cookbooks?

The meals and snacks in this book and in *The Hungry Girl Diet* were specially developed for the diet plan; they contain key ratios of fat, carbs, and protein. These recipes were also created with specific calorie and sodium limits. The Hungry Girl Diet itself was developed under the watchful eye of registered dietitian David Grotto, MS, RDN, LDN. Dave made sure that the meals and snacks in *The Hungry Girl Diet* are nutritionally sound, and these recipes were created with the same guidelines.

Where can I see photos of the recipes in this book?

Flip to the photo insert to see gorgeous, full-color photos of about fifty of these recipes! Look for the camera icon on the recipe pages to see which recipes can be found in the insert. Photos of *all* the recipes in this book can be found at hungry-girl.com/books.

A Day on the Hungry Girl Diet

Breakfast

8 ounces water

Any Breakfast from this book or *The Hungry Girl Diet*

Lunch

8 ounces water

Any Lunch/Dinner from this book or *The Hungry Girl Diet*

Dinner

8 ounces water

Any Lunch/Dinner from this book or *The Hungry Girl Diet*

Snacks

Any THREE Snacks from this book or *The Hungry Girl Diet*

8 ounces water with EACH snack

Additional Water

Have at least two more 8-ounce glasses of water throughout the day.

The Calorie Tally (and Supplemental Snacks)

It all adds up to about 1,300 calories per day. If you have 75 pounds or more to lose, have a vigorous exercise routine, or feel this calorie level is too aggressive for you, consider adding 200 calories' worth of healthy supplemental snacks to your day: fruit, veggies, lean protein, and/or nuts.

**See *The Hungry Girl Diet*
for dining-out options and
grab-n-go snacks!**

First Things First: Kitchen Staples

Here are a few essentials you'll want to have on hand . . .

Stovetop cookware:
a nonstick pot, a basic skillet, a large skillet, and a grill pan

Baking needs:
a baking sheet or two, an 8-inch by 8-inch pan, a large pan, and a 12-cup muffin pan

Microwave-safe essentials:
large mugs, bowls, and plates

Measuring must-haves:
spoons, cups, and a kitchen scale

Countertop tools:
a good blender, a meat mallet (optional), a strainer, and kitchen shears (optional, but helpful!)

HG FYI: The "measuring must-haves" may very well be the MOST important items listed here. Along with purchasing the right ingredients, *these* are how you can be sure that your meal matches the calorie count on the page. Buy 'em. Use 'em. Don't lose 'em!

Now you're ready to start whipping up HG-Diet-friendly meals and snacks . . . and dropping pounds, of course! For lots more info to help you along the way, flip to page 305 for the Go-To Guide for Grocery Shopping, Money Saving, Meal Prepping & More.

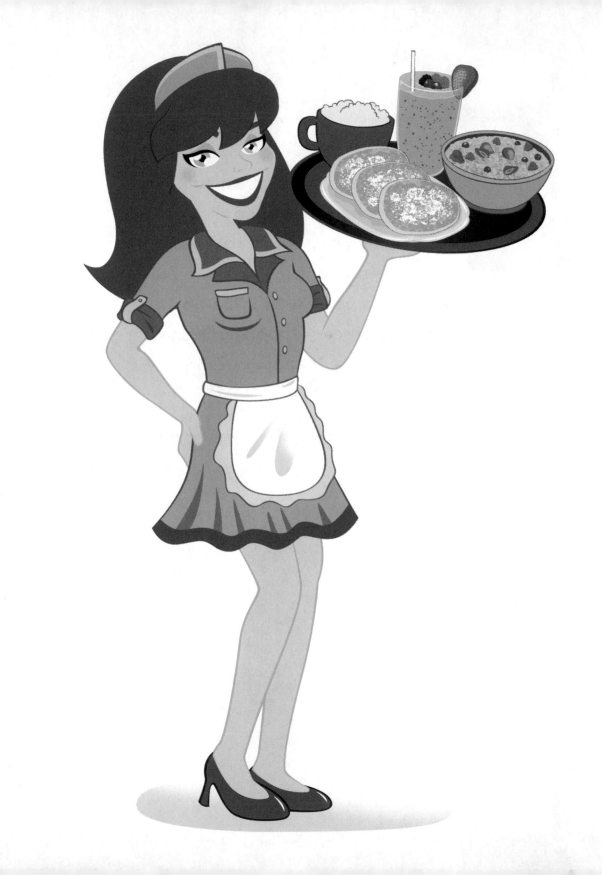

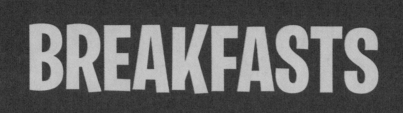

BREAKFASTS

Everything Eggs

Egg-based breakfasts are a fantastic way to start the day, especially when they're as easy, filling, and delicious as these. EggaMuffins (egg sandwiches), egg mugs (scrambles made in the microwave!), omelettes, and more . . . They're all here!

Need-to-Know Egg Mug Info!

- **You need a LARGE microwave-safe mug—the egg mixture will rise and puff as it cooks.** HG pick: a tall, wide mug with a 16-ounce capacity. No big mugs in your kitchen? Grab a sizeable microwave-safe bowl instead!

- **Don't forget to mist the mug with nonstick spray.** Spritz the sides as well as the bottom. Otherwise, some of your breakfast may stick to the mug . . .

- **Immediately after eating, soak the mug with soapy water.** This will make cleanup a snap!

- **Rather cook your scramble in a skillet?** Do it! Just spritz a skillet with nonstick spray, and cook your ingredients over medium heat, following the recipe indicators (until softened, until set, etc.).

Egg-White Assistance . . .

Using fresh whites from a shell? Here's a handy conversion chart!

¼ cup egg whites = about 2 large egg whites

⅓ cup egg whites = about 3 large egg whites

½ cup egg whites = about 4 large egg whites

Double-Cheese Veggie EggaMuffin
with berries

Entire recipe: 313 calories, 7.5g fat, 645mg sodium, 43g carbs, 14g fiber, 10.5g sugars, 23g protein

One 100-calorie flat sandwich bun or light English muffin

1 large tomato slice

1 tablespoon chopped bell pepper

1 tablespoon chopped onion

⅓ cup egg whites or fat-free liquid egg substitute

Dash garlic powder

Dash onion powder

Dash black pepper

1 wedge The Laughing Cow Light Creamy Swiss cheese

1 slice Sargento Reduced Fat Medium Cheddar cheese

1 cup raspberries and/or blackberries

You'll Need: medium microwave-safe bowl (or wide microwave-safe mug), nonstick spray

Prep: 5 minutes

Cook: 5 minutes or less

1. Toast bun/muffin halves, if you like, and top the bottom half with tomato.

2. In a medium microwave-safe bowl (or wide microwave-safe mug) sprayed with nonstick spray, microwave bell pepper and onion for 45 seconds, or until softened.

3. Add egg whites/substitute, seasonings, and cheese wedge, breaking the wedge into pieces. Mix well. Microwave for 1 minute. Gently stir and microwave for 30 seconds, or until set.

4. Transfer egg "patty" to the tomato-topped bun/muffin half.

5. Top with cheese slice and the other bun/muffin half. If you like, microwave for 15 seconds, or until cheese has melted.

6. Serve with berries.

MAKES 1 SERVING

Open-Faced Pizza EggaMuffin
with strawberries

Entire recipe: 314 calories, 6g fat, 650mg sodium, 49g carbs, 12g fiber, 16g sugars, 22g protein

One 100-calorie flat sandwich bun or light English muffin

2 tablespoons canned crushed tomatoes

2 dashes garlic powder

2 dashes onion powder

2 dashes Italian seasoning

2 tablespoons chopped onion

2 tablespoons chopped bell pepper

⅓ cup egg whites or fat-free liquid egg substitute

2 tablespoons shredded part-skim mozzarella cheese

3 slices turkey pepperoni, chopped

1 teaspoon grated Parmesan cheese

1½ cups sliced strawberries

You'll Need: microwave-safe plate, small bowl, large microwave-safe mug, nonstick spray

Prep: 5 minutes

Cook: 5 minutes or less

1. Toast bun/muffin halves, if you like, and place on a microwave-safe plate.

2. In a small bowl, stir a dash of each seasoning into crushed tomatoes. Spread onto bun/muffin halves.

3. Spray a large microwave-safe mug with nonstick spray. Microwave onion and pepper for 1½ minutes, or until softened.

4. Blot away excess moisture. Add egg whites/substitute and remaining dash of each seasoning. Mix well. Microwave for 45 seconds. Stir and microwave for another 45 seconds, or until set.

5. Divide egg scramble between bun/muffin halves. Sprinkle with mozzarella cheese, top with chopped pepperoni, and sprinkle with Parm. Microwave for 20 seconds, or until mozzarella cheese has melted and pepperoni is hot.

6. Serve with strawberries.

MAKES 1 SERVING

Turkey Cheddar EggaMuffin *with fruit*

Entire recipe: 313 calories, 8.5g fat, 530mg sodium, 37g carbs, 12g fiber, 7g sugars, 28g protein

One 100-calorie flat sandwich bun or light English muffin

½ tablespoon light whipped butter or light buttery spread

1 large tomato slice

⅓ cup egg whites or fat-free liquid egg substitute

Dash garlic powder

Dash onion powder

Dash black pepper

1 ounce (1 to 2 slices) no-salt-added turkey breast

1 slice Sargento Reduced Fat Medium Cheddar cheese

¾ cup raspberries and/or blackberries or 50 calories' worth of another fruit (page 341)

You'll Need: medium microwave-safe bowl (or wide microwave-safe mug), nonstick spray

Prep: 5 minutes

Cook: 5 minutes or less

1. Toast bun/muffin halves, if you like, and spread with butter. Top the bottom half with tomato.

2. In a medium microwave-safe bowl (or wide microwave-safe mug) sprayed with nonstick spray, combine egg whites/substitute with seasonings, and mix well. Microwave for 1 minute. Gently stir and microwave for 30 seconds, or until set.

3. Transfer egg "patty" to the tomato-topped bun/muffin half. Top with turkey, cheese, and the other bun/muffin half.

4. If you like, microwave for 15 seconds, or until cheese has melted.

5. Serve with fruit.

MAKES 1 SERVING

Guac 'n Veggie B-fast Tostada
with fruit 📷

Entire recipe: 330 calories, 7.5g fat, 590mg sodium, 50g carbs, 17g fiber, 12.5g sugars, 27g protein

1 medium-large high-fiber flour tortilla with 110 calories or less

1 ounce (about 2 tablespoons) mashed avocado

2 tablespoons fat-free plain Greek yogurt

⅛ teaspoon plus 1 dash onion powder

⅛ teaspoon plus 1 dash garlic powder

Dash chili powder

1 cup chopped spinach leaves

1 cup chopped mushrooms

½ cup chopped bell pepper

½ cup egg whites or fat-free liquid egg substitute

¼ cup seeded and diced tomato

¾ cup raspberries and/or blackberries or 50 calories' worth of another fruit (page 341)

You'll Need: baking sheet, nonstick spray, small bowl, large microwave-safe mug, medium bowl

Prep: 10 minutes

Cook: 15 minutes

1. Preheat oven to 375 degrees. Spray a baking sheet with nonstick spray.

2. Lay tortilla on the sheet, and bake until slightly crispy, about 4 minutes.

3. Flip tortilla, and bake until crispy with lightly browned edges, about 4 more minutes.

4. Meanwhile, in a small bowl, mix avocado with yogurt until uniform. Stir in a dash of each seasoning.

5. In a large microwave-safe mug, combine spinach, mushrooms, and pepper. Microwave for 2 minutes, or until softened. Transfer to a medium bowl, and blot away excess moisture.

6. Spray the mug with nonstick spray. Add egg whites/substitute and remaining ⅛ teaspoon each onion powder and garlic powder. Microwave for 1 minute. Stir and microwave for 30 seconds, or until set.

7. Spread tortilla with avocado mixture. Top with egg scramble, veggies, and tomato.

8. Serve with fruit.

MAKES 1 SERVING

📷 Photo Alert!

The camera icon next to the recipe name means flip to the insert to see a photo of this recipe. Find full-color photos of ALL the recipes at hungry-girl.com/books.

Eggs Bene-chick B-fast
with fruit

Entire recipe: 315 calories, 8g fat, 623mg sodium, 41g carbs, 8.5g fiber, 20.5g sugars, 20.5g protein

Half of a light English muffin

1½ ounces (about 3 slices) reduced-sodium ham

1 tablespoon fat-free plain Greek yogurt

1 teaspoon Dijon mustard

1 teaspoon light whipped butter or light buttery spread

1 drop lemon juice

5 asparagus spears, tough ends removed

1 teaspoon white vinegar

1 large egg

2 large tomato slices

1 cup grapefruit sections or 100 calories' worth of another fruit (page 342)

You'll Need: plate, small microwave-safe bowl, wide microwave-safe bowl, medium pot, small shallow bowl, slotted spoon

Prep: 10 minutes

Cook: 10 minutes

1. If you like, lightly toast muffin half. Top with ham, and plate muffin half.

2. To make the sauce, in a small microwave-safe bowl, combine yogurt, mustard, butter, and lemon juice. Mix until uniform.

3. Place asparagus in a wide microwave-safe bowl with 2 tablespoons water. Cover and microwave for 1 minute and 15 seconds, or until softened. Drain excess water, and cover to keep warm.

4. Fill a medium pot with 2 inches of water. Add vinegar, and bring to a boil. Once boiling, lower temperature until a steady simmer is reached.

5. Crack egg into a small shallow bowl. Give water a stir, and gently add egg. Cook until egg white is mostly opaque, 3 to 5 minutes (3 for a runnier egg, 5 for a very firm one).

6. Using a slotted spoon, carefully transfer egg to a layer of paper towels. Once excess water has been absorbed, transfer egg to the muffin half.

7. Microwave sauce until hot, about 20 seconds, and stir. (If you prefer a thinner sauce, add a bit of water.) Spoon over egg.

8. Serve with asparagus, tomato, and fruit.

MAKES 1 SERVING

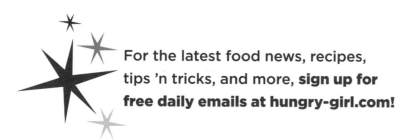

For the latest food news, recipes, tips 'n tricks, and more, **sign up for free daily emails at hungry-girl.com!**

Over-Medium Egg Sandwich
with fruit 📷

Entire recipe: 330 calories, 10g fat, 400mg sodium, 45g carbs, 10.5g fiber, 23.5g sugars, 20.5g protein

2 slices light bread

¼ cup spinach leaves

1 slice Sargento Reduced Fat Medium Cheddar cheese

1 large egg

1¼ cups orange segments or 100 calories' worth of another fruit (page 342)

Optional topping: black pepper

You'll Need: skillet, nonstick spray, microwave-safe plate (optional)

Prep: 5 minutes

Cook: 5 minutes or less

1. Toast bread, if you like, and top one slice with spinach and cheese.

2. Bring a skillet sprayed with nonstick spray to medium-low heat. Cook egg until white is fully cooked and yolk is mostly cooked, 1 to 2 minutes per side, flipping carefully.

3. If you like, place cheese-topped bread slice on a microwave-safe plate, and microwave for 15 seconds, or until cheese has melted. Top with egg and the other bread slice.

4. Serve with fruit.

MAKES 1 SERVING

Top Turkey Egg Mug
with bun and berries

Entire recipe: 310 calories, 6g fat, 646mg sodium, 38g carbs, 12g fiber, 8g sugars, 28.5g protein

One 100-calorie flat sandwich bun or light English muffin

½ tablespoon light whipped butter or light buttery spread

½ cup egg whites or fat-free liquid egg substitute

⅛ teaspoon onion powder

⅛ teaspoon garlic powder

Dash black pepper

1 ounce (1 to 2 slices) chopped no-salt-added turkey breast

2 tablespoons seeded and diced tomato

1 wedge The Laughing Cow Light Creamy Swiss cheese

¾ cup raspberries and/or blackberries

You'll Need: large microwave-safe mug, nonstick spray

Prep: 5 minutes

Cook: 5 minutes or less

1. Toast bun/muffin halves, if you like, and spread with butter.

2. Spray a large microwave-safe mug with nonstick spray. Add egg whites/substitute and seasonings. Stir, and microwave for 1 minute.

3. Stir in turkey, tomato, and cheese wedge, breaking the wedge into pieces. Microwave for 1 more minute, or until set.

4. Serve with berries and buttered bun/muffin.

MAKES 1 SERVING

Chicken Feta Egg Mug
with bun and fruit 📷

Entire recipe: 327 calories, 6g fat, 625mg sodium, 44g carbs, 13.5g fiber, 11.5g sugars, 29g protein

One 100-calorie flat sandwich bun or light English muffin

½ tablespoon light whipped butter or light buttery spread

½ cup egg whites or fat-free liquid egg substitute

2 tablespoons finely chopped bagged sun-dried tomatoes

⅛ teaspoon onion powder

⅛ teaspoon garlic powder

Dash black pepper, or more for topping

1 ounce cooked and chopped skinless chicken breast

1 tablespoon crumbled reduced-fat feta cheese

½ tablespoon chopped fresh basil

¾ cup raspberries and/or blackberries or 50 calories' worth of another fruit (page 341)

You'll Need: large microwave-safe mug, nonstick spray

Prep: 5 minutes

Cook: 5 minutes or less

1. Toast bun/muffin halves, if you like, and spread with butter.

2. In a large microwave-safe mug sprayed with nonstick spray, combine egg whites/substitute, sun-dried tomatoes, and seasonings. Mix well, and microwave for 1 minute.

3. Stir in chicken, cheese, and basil. Microwave for 1 minute, or until set.

4. Serve with fruit and buttered bun/muffin.

MAKES 1 SERVING

HG Alternative

If you can only find sun-dried tomatoes that are packed in oil, drain and rinse them really well, and then pat dry. This will get rid of excess fat.

Open-Faced Avocado EggaMuffin *with fruit*

Entire recipe: 319 calories, 8.5g fat, 642mg sodium, 41g carbs, 14g fiber, 9g sugars, 21.5g protein

One 100-calorie flat sandwich bun or light English muffin

½ tablespoon light whipped butter or light buttery spread

2 large tomato slices

¾ ounce thinly sliced avocado (about ⅛ of an avocado)

½ cup chopped spinach leaves

½ cup egg whites or fat-free liquid egg substitute

⅛ teaspoon onion powder

⅛ teaspoon garlic powder

Dash black pepper

1 wedge The Laughing Cow Light Creamy Swiss cheese

¾ cup raspberries and/or blackberries or 50 calories' worth of another fruit (page 341)

You'll Need: large microwave-safe mug, nonstick spray

Prep: 5 minutes

Cook: 5 minutes or less

1. Toast bun/muffin halves, if you like, and spread with butter.

2. Top each half with a tomato slice, and evenly divide avocado between the halves.

3. In a large microwave-safe mug sprayed with nonstick spray, microwave spinach for 30 seconds, or until wilted.

4. Blot away excess moisture. Add egg whites/substitute and seasonings, stir, and microwave for 1 minute.

5. Mix in cheese wedge, breaking it into pieces. Microwave for 1 more minute, or until set.

6. Evenly top bun/muffin halves with egg scramble.

7. Serve with fruit.

MAKES 1 SERVING

Black Bean 'n Cheese Egg Mug
with bun and fruit

Entire recipe: 326 calories, 7.5g fat, 619mg sodium, 45.5g carbs, 14g fiber, 9g sugars, 24.5g protein

One 100-calorie flat sandwich bun or light English muffin

½ tablespoon light whipped butter or light buttery spread

¼ cup chopped bell pepper

2 tablespoons chopped onion

½ cup egg whites or fat-free liquid egg substitute

⅛ teaspoon onion powder

⅛ teaspoon garlic powder

Dash chili powder

Dash ground cumin

2 tablespoons shredded reduced-fat cheddar cheese

2 tablespoons canned black beans, drained and rinsed

¾ cup raspberries and/or blackberries or 50 calories' worth of another fruit (page 341)

You'll Need: large microwave-safe mug, nonstick spray

Prep: 5 minutes

Cook: 5 minutes or less

1. Toast bun/muffin halves, if you like, and spread with butter.

2. In a large microwave-safe mug sprayed with nonstick spray, microwave pepper and onion for 1½ minutes, or until softened.

3. Blot away excess moisture. Add egg whites/substitute and seasonings, stir, and microwave for 1 minute.

4. Stir in cheese and beans. Microwave for 45 seconds, or until set.

5. Serve with fruit and buttered bun/muffin.

MAKES 1 SERVING

Open-Faced Caprese EggaMuffin
with strawberries

Entire recipe: 324 calories, 9g fat, 494mg sodium, 43.5g carbs, 10.5g fiber, 13g sugars, 23g protein

One 100-calorie flat sandwich bun or light English muffin

2 large tomato slices

½ cup egg whites or fat-free liquid egg substitute

2 tablespoons shredded part-skim mozzarella cheese

1 tablespoon finely chopped fresh basil

1 teaspoon extra-virgin olive oil

1½ cups strawberries

You'll Need: large microwave-safe mug, nonstick spray

Prep: 5 minutes

Cook: 5 minutes or less

1. Toast bun/muffin halves, if you like. Top each half with a tomato slice.

2. In a large microwave-safe mug sprayed with nonstick spray, microwave egg whites/substitute for 1 minute.

3. Stir in cheese, and microwave for 1 more minute, or until set.

4. Divide egg mixture between bun/muffin halves, sprinkle with basil, and drizzle with olive oil.

5. Serve with strawberries.

MAKES 1 SERVING

Cheesed-Up Spinach B-fast Tostada
with orange segments

Entire recipe: 312 calories, 6g fat, 618mg sodium, 38.5g carbs, 7.5g fiber, 19.5g sugars, 23g protein

1 teaspoon light whipped butter or light buttery spread

One 6-inch corn tortilla

2 cups chopped spinach leaves

2 teaspoons grated Parmesan cheese

¼ teaspoon garlic powder

1 wedge The Laughing Cow Light Creamy Swiss cheese

½ cup egg whites or fat-free liquid egg substitute

2 tablespoons finely chopped bagged sun-dried tomatoes

¾ cup orange segments

You'll Need: skillet, plate, medium microwave-safe bowl, nonstick spray

Prep: 5 minutes

Cook: 10 minutes

1. Bring a skillet to medium-high heat. Add butter, and let it coat the bottom. Cook tortilla until lightly browned, about 2 minutes per side. Transfer to a plate.

2. In a medium microwave-safe bowl, microwave spinach for 30 seconds, or until wilted. Blot away excess moisture. Add Parmesan cheese, ⅛ teaspoon garlic powder, and cheese wedge, breaking the wedge into pieces. Mix thoroughly.

3. Spread mixture onto the tortilla.

4. Spray skillet with nonstick spray, and bring to medium heat. Add egg whites/substitute, sun-dried tomatoes, and remaining ⅛ teaspoon garlic powder. Cook and scramble for about 2 minutes, until fully cooked.

5. Place scramble over the loaded tostada, and serve with orange segments.

MAKES 1 SERVING

HG Alternative

If you can only find sun-dried tomatoes that are packed in oil, drain and rinse them really well, and then pat dry. This will get rid of excess fat.

Half 'n Half Scramble
with fruit

Entire recipe: 330 calories, 9g fat, 580mg sodium, 38g carbs, 4.5g fiber, 23.5g sugars, 27.5 protein

1 large egg

½ cup egg whites or fat-free liquid egg substitute

⅛ teaspoon garlic powder

⅛ teaspoon black pepper

⅔ cup chopped mushrooms

⅔ cup chopped bell pepper

⅔ cup chopped onion

2½ tablespoons shredded reduced-fat Mexican-blend cheese

3 tablespoons salsa or pico de gallo with 90mg sodium or less per 2-tablespoon serving

½ cup grapes or 50 calories' worth of another fruit (page 341)

You'll Need: medium-large bowl, whisk, large skillet with a lid, nonstick spray

Prep: 5 minutes

Cook: 10 minutes

1. In a medium-large bowl, combine egg, egg whites/substitute, garlic powder, and black pepper. Whisk thoroughly.

2. Bring a large skillet sprayed with nonstick spray to medium heat. Add mushrooms, bell pepper, and onion. Cook and stir until softened and lightly browned, about 4 minutes.

3. Reduce heat to medium low, and add egg mixture to the skillet. Cook and scramble for about 4 minutes, until fully cooked.

4. Remove from heat, and stir in cheese.

5. Serve topped with salsa/pico de gallo and alongside fruit.

MAKES 1 SERVING

Breakfast Soft Tacos 📷

Entire recipe: 318 calories, 6g fat, 615mg sodium, 36g carbs, 6g fiber, 4g sugars, 28.5g protein

2 tablespoons chopped onion

⅔ cup egg whites or fat-free liquid egg substitute

Dash garlic powder

Dash chili powder

Dash black pepper

¼ cup canned black beans, drained and rinsed

3 tablespoons shredded reduced-fat Mexican-blend cheese

Two 6-inch corn tortillas

¼ cup chopped tomato

You'll Need: large microwave-safe mug, nonstick spray, microwave-safe plate

Prep: 5 minutes

Cook: 5 minutes or less

1. In a large microwave-safe mug sprayed with nonstick spray, microwave onion until soft, about 1 minute.

2. Add egg whites/substitute and seasonings. Microwave for 1 minute. Stir in black beans, and microwave for 30 seconds, or until egg is set. Stir in cheese.

3. Microwave tortillas on a microwave-safe plate for 10 seconds, or until warm. Evenly divide egg mixture between the centers of the tortillas. Top with tomato, and fold 'em up.

MAKES 1 SERVING

Open-Faced Poached EggaMuffin *with fruit*

Entire recipe: 327 calories, 10.5g fat, 520mg sodium, 45g carbs, 11g fiber, 14.5g sugars, 20.5g protein

1 light English muffin

2 large tomato slices

1 teaspoon white vinegar

2 large eggs

2 cups spinach leaves

⅛ teaspoon garlic powder

⅛ teaspoon onion powder

Dash salt

3 dashes black pepper

⅔ cup orange segments or 50 calories' worth of another fruit (page 341)

You'll Need: plate, medium pot, small shallow bowl, slotted spoon, skillet, nonstick spray

Prep: 5 minutes

Cook: 20 minutes

1. Toast bun/muffin halves, if you like, and top each half with a tomato slice. Plate muffin halves.

2. Fill a medium pot with 2 inches of water. Add vinegar, and bring to a boil. Once boiling, lower temperature until a steady simmer is reached.

3. Crack one egg into a small shallow bowl. Give water a stir, and gently add egg. Cook until egg white is mostly opaque, 3 to 5 minutes (3 for a runnier egg, 5 for very firm one).

4. Using a slotted spoon, carefully transfer egg to a layer of paper towels to absorb excess water. Repeat process with remaining egg.

5. Bring a skillet sprayed with nonstick spray to medium-high heat. Add spinach, garlic powder, onion powder, salt, and a dash of pepper. Cook and stir until wilted, about 2 minutes.

6. Evenly divide spinach between muffin halves. Top each muffin half with a poached egg and a dash of pepper.

7. Serve with fruit.

MAKES 1 SERVING

Portabella Poached Egg
with fruit-topped yogurt 📷

Entire recipe: 323 calories, 9g fat, 496mg sodium, 38.5g carbs, 5g fiber, 29g sugars, 23.5g protein

1 portabella mushroom cap (stem removed)

1 cup spinach leaves

Dash salt

1 teaspoon white vinegar

1 large egg

1 slice Sargento Reduced Fat Medium Cheddar cheese

1 large tomato slice

6 ounces (about ¾ cup) fat-free vanilla yogurt

½ cup chopped apple

Optional: black pepper

You'll Need: baking sheet, nonstick spray, medium pot, small shallow bowl, slotted spoon, plate, medium bowl

Prep: 10 minutes

Cook: 20 minutes

1. Preheat oven to 400 degrees. Spray a baking sheet with nonstick spray.

2. Place mushroom cap on the sheet, rounded side down. Bake until tender, about 15 minutes. Remove sheet, but leave oven on.

3. Meanwhile, bring a medium pot sprayed with nonstick spray to medium-high heat. Add spinach and salt. Cook and stir until wilted, about 1 minute. Remove from heat, and blot away excess moisture.

4. Clean pot, and fill with 2 inches of water. Add vinegar, and bring to a boil. Once boiling, lower temperature until a steady simmer is reached.

5. Crack egg into a small shallow bowl. Give water a stir, and gently add egg. Cook until egg white is mostly opaque, 3 to 5 minutes (3 for a runnier egg, 5 for a very firm one).

6. Using a slotted spoon, carefully transfer egg to a layer of paper towels to absorb excess water.

7. Blot excess moisture from mushroom cap, and top with cheese slice. Bake until cheese begins to melt, 1 to 2 minutes. Transfer to a plate, and top with tomato, spinach, and egg. If you like, sprinkle with black pepper.

8. In a medium bowl, top yogurt with apple. Serve with egg-topped portabella.

MAKES 1 SERVING

Strawberry Stuffed Omelette
with PB-topped English muffin

Entire recipe: 326 calories, 7.5g fat, 576mg sodium, 32.5g carbs, 6g fiber, 13g sugars, 32g protein

Half of a 100-calorie sandwich bun or light English muffin

2½ teaspoons creamy peanut butter

¾ cup sliced strawberries

⅛ teaspoon cinnamon

1 tablespoon low-sugar strawberry preserves

1 cup egg whites or fat-free liquid egg substitute

You'll Need: medium bowl, medium skillet with a lid, nonstick spray, plate

Prep: 5 minutes

Cook: 5 minutes

1. Toast bun/muffin half, if you like, and spread with peanut butter.

2. In a medium bowl, sprinkle strawberries with cinnamon. Add preserves, and stir to coat.

3. Bring a medium skillet sprayed with nonstick spray to medium-low heat. Add egg whites/substitute, and let it coat the bottom of the skillet.

4. Cover and cook without stirring for 3 minutes, or until just set.

5. Evenly distribute strawberry mixture onto one half of the omelette. Fold the bare half over the filling, and slide your stuffed omelette onto a plate. Serve with PB-topped bun/muffin half.

MAKES 1 SERVING

Growing Oatmeal, Oat Bran, Quinoa & More

Growing oatmeal is a staple on the Hungry Girl Diet (and in the HG world, in general!). That's because it allows you to enjoy a HUGE bowl of creamy oatmeal without consuming a lot of calories. The trick is to cook it for twice as long as ordinary oatmeal, using twice as much liquid. And for the first time ever, we're whipping up growing oat bran too!

Growing Oatmeal 101

What is it? Super-sized hot cereal! Compared to standard old-fashioned oatmeal, HG growing oatmeal calls for twice as much liquid—part milk for creaminess; part water to keep calorie counts down. It also cooks for twice as long, so the extra liquid is absorbed and the oats really puff up. The result? A super-large breakfast bowl *without* a super-large calorie count!

Why fat-free milk? One word: PROTEIN. Swaps like unsweetened almond milk and light soymilk are fantastic, but those generally don't have as much protein as dairy milk. And the oatmeal bowls on the Hungry Girl Diet need that protein to make them extra filling and perfectly balanced. Can't do dairy? Go for lactose-free nonfat milk.

Why old-fashioned oats? Simple. The long cook time is key when making the oatmeal grow. And if you cooked instant or five-minute oats for that long, they'd turn to mush.

Will it thicken? YES. Although it looks like a lot of liquid, and hasn't completely thickened once it's done cooking, it *will* thicken after you've transferred it to a bowl. Give it 5 to 10 minutes; you'll see!

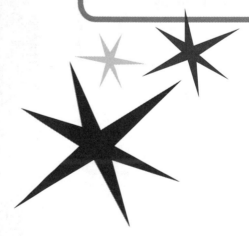

Banana-mon Oatmeal
with hard-boiled egg whites

Entire recipe: 330 calories, 6g fat, 419mg sodium, 48g carbs, 5.5g fiber, 16g sugars, 19g protein

½ cup old-fashioned oats

¼ teaspoon cinnamon

⅛ teaspoon vanilla extract

Dash salt

¾ cup fat-free milk

3 tablespoons mashed ripe banana

2 teaspoons light whipped butter or light buttery spread

1 no-calorie sweetener packet

2 large hard-boiled egg whites

You'll Need: nonstick pot, medium bowl

Prep: 5 minutes

Cook: 20 minutes

1. In a nonstick pot, combine oats, cinnamon, vanilla extract, salt, and milk.

2. Mix in 1¼ cups water. Bring to a boil, and then reduce to a simmer.

3. Add banana, and cook and stir until thick and creamy, 12 to 15 minutes.

4. Transfer to a medium bowl, and stir in butter and sweetener. Let cool until thickened.

5. Serve with egg whites.

MAKES 1 SERVING

Peaches 'n Cream Oatmeal 📷

Entire recipe: 326 calories, 6.5g fat, 271mg sodium, 49g carbs, 5.5g fiber, 18.5g sugars, 18.5g protein

½ cup old-fashioned oats

¼ teaspoon cinnamon

⅛ teaspoon vanilla extract

Dash salt

¾ cup fat-free milk

¼ cup chopped peaches (fresh or thawed from frozen)

1 no-calorie sweetener packet

¼ cup fat-free peach Greek yogurt

¼ ounce (about 1 tablespoon) sliced almonds

You'll Need: nonstick pot, medium bowl

Prep: 5 minutes

Cook: 20 minutes

1. In a nonstick pot, combine oats, cinnamon, vanilla extract, salt, and milk.

2. Mix in 1¼ cups water. Bring to a boil, and then reduce to a simmer.

3. Add peaches, and cook and stir until thick and creamy, 12 to 15 minutes.

4. Transfer to a medium bowl, and stir in sweetener. Let cool until thickened.

5. Top with yogurt and almonds.

MAKES 1 SERVING

No-Cal Sweetener Newsflash!

Packets of calorie-free sweetener come in *so* many varieties, including stevia-based kinds and other all-natural picks. Choose your favorite!

Pineapple Coconut Oatmeal
with hard-boiled egg whites

Entire recipe: 330 calories, 6.5g fat, 406mg sodium, 46.5g carbs, 6g fiber, 16.5g sugars, 20g protein

½ cup old-fashioned oats

¼ teaspoon cinnamon

⅛ teaspoon vanilla extract

Dash salt

⅔ cup fat-free milk

1 no-calorie sweetener packet

3 tablespoons chopped pineapple

1 tablespoon sweetened shredded coconut

1 tablespoon fat-free vanilla Greek yogurt

2 large hard-boiled egg whites

You'll Need: nonstick pot, medium bowl

Prep: 5 minutes

Cook: 20 minutes

1. In a nonstick pot, combine oats, cinnamon, vanilla extract, salt, and milk.

2. Mix in 1¼ cups water. Bring to a boil, and then reduce to a simmer.

3. Cook and stir until thick and creamy, 12 to 15 minutes.

4. Transfer to a medium bowl, and stir in sweetener. Let cool until thickened.

5. Top with pineapple, coconut, and yogurt, and serve with egg whites.

MAKES 1 SERVING

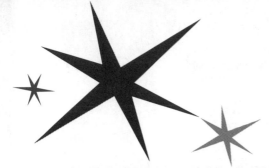

Grow Your Oatmeal in the Microwave!

Heads up: You need a REALLY big bowl . . .

1. Mix your main ingredients as usual, but in a microwave-safe bowl with at least a 10-cup capacity. (You read that right. The oatmeal bubbles up A LOT in the microwave.)

2. Cover and microwave for 12 to 15 minutes, until thick and creamy, stirring halfway through.

3. Stir in any remaining ingredients, and let cool to thicken. Tada!

Pear 'n Pistachio Oatmeal
with hard-boiled egg whites

Entire recipe: 323 calories, 6.5g fat, 362mg sodium, 46.5g carbs, 6g fiber, 15g sugars, 21g protein

½ cup old-fashioned oats

¼ cup peeled and chopped pear

¼ teaspoon cinnamon

⅛ teaspoon nutmeg

⅛ teaspoon vanilla extract

Dash salt

¾ cup fat-free milk

1 no-calorie sweetener packet

¼ ounce (about 1 tablespoon) chopped pistachios

2 large hard-boiled egg whites

You'll Need: nonstick pot, medium bowl

Prep: 5 minutes

Cook: 20 minutes

1. In a nonstick pot, combine oats, pear, cinnamon, nutmeg, vanilla extract, salt, and milk.

2. Mix in 1¼ cups water. Bring to a boil, and then reduce to a simmer.

3. Cook and stir until thick and creamy, 12 to 15 minutes.

4. Transfer to a medium bowl, and stir in sweetener. Let cool until thickened.

5. Top with pistachios, and serve with egg whites.

MAKES 1 SERVING

Hard-Boiled Advice!

For a step-by-step guide to hard-boiling egg whites—plus a super list of swaps—flip to page 323!

Raspberry White Chocolate Oatmeal
with hard-boiled egg whites

Entire recipe: 321 calories, 5.5g fat, 369mg sodium, 47.5g carbs, 7g fiber, 17g sugars, 20g protein

½ cup old-fashioned oats

¼ teaspoon cinnamon

⅛ teaspoon vanilla extract

Dash salt

¾ cup fat-free milk

1 no-calorie sweetener packet

⅓ cup raspberries

1½ teaspoons white chocolate chips, chopped

2 large hard-boiled egg whites

You'll Need: nonstick pot, medium bowl

Prep: 5 minutes

Cook: 20 minutes

1. In a nonstick pot, combine oats, cinnamon, vanilla extract, salt, and milk.

2. Mix in 1¼ cups water. Bring to a boil, and then reduce to a simmer.

3. Cook and stir until thick and creamy, 12 to 15 minutes.

4. Transfer to a medium bowl, and stir in sweetener. Let cool until thickened.

5. Top with berries and white chocolate chips, and serve with egg whites.

MAKES 1 SERVING

Overnight Oatmeal

Entire recipe: 330 calories, 7.5g fat, 229mg sodium, 47.5g carbs, 7.5g fiber, 16g sugars, 20.5g protein

½ cup old-fashioned oats

½ cup fat-free vanilla Greek yogurt

¼ cup fat-free milk

⅛ teaspoon cinnamon

1 no-calorie sweetener packet

Dash salt

1 drop vanilla extract

¼ cup blackberries and/or raspberries

⅓ ounce (about 1½ tablespoons) sliced almonds or chopped pistachios

You'll Need: medium jar or bowl

Prep: 10 minutes

Chill: 8 hours or more

1. In a medium jar or bowl, combine all ingredients *except* berries and nuts.

2. Cover and refrigerate for at least 8 hours, until oats are soft and have absorbed most of the liquid.

3. Stir oatmeal. Top with berries and nuts.

MAKES 1 SERVING

Overnight Oatmeal Parfait 📷

Entire recipe: 324 calories, 8g fat, 252mg sodium, 45g carbs, 7g fiber, 12.5g sugars, 21g protein

¼ cup unsweetened vanilla almond milk

2 tablespoons vanilla protein powder with about 100 calories per serving

½ cup old-fashioned oats

1 no-calorie sweetener packet

⅛ teaspoon cinnamon

1 drop vanilla extract

Dash salt

⅓ cup fat-free vanilla Greek yogurt

½ cup sliced strawberries

¼ ounce (about 1 tablespoon) sliced almonds or chopped pistachios

You'll Need: medium bowl, mid-sized glass

Prep: 10 minutes

Chill: 8 hours

1. In a medium bowl, combine almond milk, protein powder, oats, sweetener, cinnamon, vanilla extract, and salt. Mix well.

2. Cover and refrigerate for at least 8 hours, until oats are soft and have absorbed most of the liquid.

3. Stir oatmeal. In a mid-sized glass, layer half of each ingredient: oatmeal, yogurt, and strawberries.

4. Repeat layering with remaining oatmeal, yogurt, and strawberries. Top with nuts.

MAKES 1 SERVING

Zucchini Walnut Oat Bran

Entire recipe: 320 calories, 8g fat, 373mg sodium, 41g carbs, 9.5g fiber, 16.5g sugars, 21g protein

½ cup shredded zucchini

¼ cup oat bran

1 teaspoon chia seeds

¼ teaspoon cinnamon

⅛ teaspoon vanilla extract

Dash salt

1 cup fat-free milk

¼ cup canned pure pumpkin

3 tablespoons liquid egg whites

1 no-calorie sweetener packet

¼ ounce (about 1 tablespoon) chopped walnuts

You'll Need: nonstick pot, medium bowl

Prep: 5 minutes

Cook: 10 minutes

1. In a nonstick pot, combine zucchini, oat bran, chia seeds, cinnamon, vanilla extract, salt, and milk.

2. Mix in ½ cup water. Bring to a boil, and then reduce heat to low.

3. Add pumpkin, and mix well. Stirring continuously, gradually add egg whites. Cook and stir until thick and creamy, about 6 minutes.

4. Transfer to a medium bowl, and stir in sweetener. Let cool until thickened.

5. Top with walnuts.

MAKES 1 SERVING

Ch-Ch-Ch-Chia!

Go ahead, get all the Chia Pet jokes out of your system . . . Chia seeds are full of good stuff: fiber, protein, omega-3s, and more. Plus, they expand when added to liquid, so eating them can help you feel full. They're fantastic in these recipes—try 'em!

Apple Cinnamon Oat Bran
with hard-boiled egg whites

Entire recipe: 323 calories, 6g fat, 362mg sodium, 46.5g carbs, 13g fiber, 19g sugars, 22g protein

¼ cup oat bran

1 tablespoon chia seeds

¼ teaspoon plus
⅛ teaspoon cinnamon

⅛ teaspoon vanilla extract

Dash salt

¾ cup fat-free milk

¼ cup canned pure pumpkin

½ cup chopped apple

1 no-calorie sweetener packet

2 large hard-boiled egg whites

You'll Need: nonstick pot, medium bowl

Prep: 5 minutes

Cook: 15 minutes

1. In a nonstick pot, combine oat bran, chia seeds, cinnamon, vanilla extract, salt, and milk.

2. Mix in ¾ cup water. Bring to a boil, and then reduce to a simmer.

3. Add pumpkin and apple. Cook and stir until thick and creamy, 6 to 8 minutes.

4. Transfer to a medium bowl, and stir in sweetener. Let cool until thickened.

5. Serve with egg whites.

MAKES 1 SERVING

Why Pumpkin?

Don't worry; it won't make your breakfast taste like Thanksgiving. It just adds creaminess and brings a fiber boost. Even if you don't like the taste of pumpkin, you should totally give this a try . . .

Strawberry Pistachio Quinoa 📷

Entire recipe: 310 calories, 6g fat, 323mg sodium, 44.5g carbs, 5g fiber, 11g sugars, 18g protein

¼ cup uncooked quinoa, thoroughly rinsed

⅛ teaspoon cinnamon

⅛ teaspoon vanilla extract

Dash salt

½ cup fat-free milk

¼ cup liquid egg whites

1 no-calorie sweetener packet

⅓ cup chopped strawberries

¼ ounce (about 1 tablespoon) chopped pistachios

You'll Need: nonstick pot, medium bowl

Prep: 5 minutes

Cook: 20 minutes

1. In a nonstick pot, combine quinoa, cinnamon, vanilla extract, salt, and milk.

2. Mix in 1 cup water. Bring to a boil, and then reduce to a simmer.

3. Stirring continuously, gradually add egg whites. Cook and stir until thick and creamy, 14 to 16 minutes.

4. Transfer to a medium bowl, and stir in sweetener. Let cool until thickened.

5. Top with strawberries and pistachios.

MAKES 1 SERVING

📷 Photo Alert!

The camera icon next to the recipe name means flip to the insert to see a photo of this recipe. Find full-color photos of ALL the recipes at hungry-girl.com/books.

Quinoa Queries!

Why is there egg in this hot cereal?

While oats and oat bran expand when you add liquid, quinoa doesn't work quite the same way. Stirring liquid egg whites into the mixture while it cooks gives you a slightly larger serving with added creaminess and a nice protein boost! Plus, it tastes GREAT!

Not into this at all? Just have a side of two hard-boiled egg whites instead. See Super Swaps for Hard-Boiled Egg Whites on page 324 for more options!

Why do I need to rinse the quinoa?

Rinsing rids the grain of its slightly bitter coating. It also removes any inedible particles that tend to pop up in whole grains. Use a fine mesh strainer, or buy pre-rinsed quinoa.

Cherry Almond Quinoa

Entire recipe: 318 calories, 6g fat, 324mg sodium, 45.5g carbs, 5g fiber, 12.5g sugars, 18g protein

¼ cup uncooked quinoa, thoroughly rinsed

¼ teaspoon cinnamon

⅛ teaspoon vanilla extract

Dash salt

½ cup fat-free milk

¼ cup liquid egg whites

1 no-calorie sweetener packet

¼ cup unsweetened pitted dark sweet cherries (fresh or thawed from frozen and drained), chopped

¼ ounce (about 1 tablespoon) sliced almonds

You'll Need: nonstick pot, medium bowl

Prep: 5 minutes

Cook: 20 minutes

1. In a nonstick pot, combine quinoa, cinnamon, vanilla extract, salt, and milk.

2. Mix in 1 cup water. Bring to a boil, and then reduce to a simmer.

3. Stirring continuously, gradually add egg whites. Cook and stir until thick and creamy, 14 to 16 minutes.

4. Transfer to a medium bowl, and stir in sweetener. Let cool until thickened.

5. Top with chopped cherries and almonds.

MAKES 1 SERVING

Supercharged Cereal Bowl

Entire recipe: 330 calories, 7.5g fat, 234mg sodium, 61g carbs, 20.5g fiber, 7g sugars, 19.5g protein

1 cup light vanilla soymilk

2 tablespoons vanilla protein powder with about 100 calories per serving

½ cup puffed rice cereal

½ cup unfrosted bite-sized shredded wheat cereal

½ cup Fiber One Original bran cereal

¼ cup raspberries

¼ ounce (about 1 tablespoon) sliced almonds

You'll Need: medium bowl, whisk

Prep: 5 minutes

1. Pour soymilk into a medium bowl. Add protein powder, and whisk to dissolve.

2. Add remaining ingredients.

MAKES 1 SERVING

For the latest food news, recipes, tips 'n tricks, and more, **sign up for free daily emails at hungry-girl.com!**

Protein-Packed Fruit Bowls & Breakfast Smoothies

Fruit is so filling, especially when it's paired with high-protein Greek yogurt and other nutritious ingredients. These breakfasts are perfect when you're in a rush, on the go, or just craving some fruity goodness . . .

Peach Mango Bowl

Entire recipe: 323 calories, 7.5g fat, 124mg sodium, 53g carbs, 12.5g fiber, 32g sugars, 23.5g protein

6 ounces (about ⅔ cup) fat-free plain Greek yogurt

1 no-calorie sweetener packet

Dash cinnamon

1 cup chopped peach (fresh or thawed from frozen)

½ cup chopped mango (fresh or thawed from frozen)

¼ cup Fiber One Original bran cereal

½ ounce (about 2 tablespoons) chopped pistachios

You'll Need: medium bowl

Prep: 5 minutes

In a medium bowl, mix sweetener and cinnamon into yogurt. Top with remaining ingredients.

MAKES 1 SERVING

Why Greek Yogurt?

It has around TWICE as much protein as regular yogurt, which makes it more filling. Plus, it's thick, creamy, and delicious. Think plain Greek yogurt is too tart for your taste buds? The sweetener in these recipes makes it *perfect*.

Mega Mint 'n Melon Bowl

Entire recipe: 315 calories, 8.5g fat, 150mg sodium, 48.5g carbs, 11g fiber, 29g sugars, 24g protein

6 ounces (about ⅔ cup) fat-free plain Greek yogurt

1 no-calorie sweetener packet

1 cup cubed watermelon

1 cup cubed cantaloupe

1 tablespoon chopped mint leaves

¼ cup Fiber One Original bran cereal

½ ounce (about 2 tablespoons) sliced almonds

You'll Need: small bowl, medium-large bowl

Prep: 5 minutes

1. In a small bowl, stir sweetener into yogurt.

2. In a medium-large bowl, toss watermelon, cantaloupe, and mint. Top with sweetened yogurt, cereal, and almonds.

MAKES 1 SERVING

Fiber One Alternatives

I love Fiber One Original bran cereal: only 60 calories per ½-cup serving, plus 14 grams of fiber! But if you avoid aspartame, you've got options: **Nature's Path Organic SmartBran** and **All-Bran Original.**

Each of these alternatives has an additional 20 calories per ½ cup; the SmartBran has one less gram of fiber, and the All-Bran has four fewer. However, since most of the bran-cereal recipes in this book call for ¼ cup or less, the differences are fairly negligible.

PB&J Bowl

Entire recipe: 310 calories, 9g fat, 190mg sodium, 43g carbs, 13g fiber, 19.5g sugars, 24g protein

6 ounces (about ⅔ cup) fat-free plain Greek yogurt

1 tablespoon creamy peanut butter

1 no-calorie sweetener packet

Dash cinnamon

1½ cups chopped strawberries

¼ cup Fiber One Original bran cereal

You'll Need: medium bowl

Prep: 5 minutes

1. In a medium bowl, combine yogurt, peanut butter, sweetener, and cinnamon. Mix until uniform.

2. Top with strawberries and cereal.

MAKES 1 SERVING

Pineapple Grape Bowl

Entire recipe: 325 calories, 6.5g fat, 73mg sodium, 49.5g carbs, 7g fiber, 36.5g sugars, 22.5g protein

6 ounces (about ⅔ cup) fat-free plain Greek yogurt

2 teaspoons chia seeds

¼ teaspoon cinnamon

1 no-calorie sweetener packet

¾ cup chopped pineapple

¾ cup halved grapes

¼ ounce (about 1 tablespoon) sliced almonds

You'll Need: medium bowl

Prep: 5 minutes

---

1. In a medium bowl, combine yogurt, chia seeds, cinnamon, and sweetener. Mix well.

2. Top with remaining ingredients.

MAKES 1 SERVING

No-Cal Sweetener Newsflash!

Packets of calorie-free sweetener come in *so* many varieties, including stevia-based kinds and other all-natural picks. Choose your favorite!

Apple Cinnamon Bowl

Entire recipe: 323 calories, 9g fat, 454mg sodium, 41g carbs, 7.5g fiber, 28.5g sugars, 22g protein

½ cup 2% low-fat cottage cheese

¼ cup fat-free plain Greek yogurt

1½ teaspoons chia seeds

¼ teaspoon cinnamon

1 no-calorie sweetener packet

1¼ cups chopped apple

1 tablespoon raisins, chopped

¼ ounce (about 1 tablespoon) chopped walnuts

You'll Need: medium bowl

Prep: 5 minutes

1. In a medium bowl, combine cottage cheese, yogurt, chia seeds, cinnamon, and sweetener. Mix well.

2. Top with remaining ingredients.

MAKES 1 SERVING

Triple Berry Bowl
with English muffin

Entire recipe: 316 calories, 9g fat, 549mg sodium, 46.5g carbs, 15.5g fiber, 17.5g sugars, 20g protein

Half of a light English muffin

1 teaspoon light whipped butter or light buttery spread

½ cup 2% low-fat cottage cheese

1 no-calorie sweetener packet

1 drop vanilla extract

⅔ cup raspberries

⅔ cup blackberries

⅓ cup blueberries

¼ ounce (about 1 tablespoon) sliced almonds

You'll Need: small bowl, medium bowl

Prep: 5 minutes

1. If you like, lightly toast muffin half. Spread with butter.

2. In a small bowl, combine cottage cheese, sweetener, and vanilla extract. Mix well.

3. Place berries in a medium bowl. Top with cottage cheese mixture and almonds, and serve with buttered muffin half.

MAKES 1 SERVING

Peach Almond Smoothie

Entire recipe: 325 calories, 9.5g fat, 141mg sodium, 42g carbs, 5.5g fiber, 31g sugars, 23.5g protein

1⅔ cups frozen unsweetened peach slices, partially thawed

¾ cup fat-free milk

¼ cup vanilla protein powder with about 100 calories per serving

1 tablespoon almond butter

1½ cups crushed ice *or* 8 to 12 ice cubes

You'll Need: blender

Prep: 5 minutes

Place all ingredients in a blender. Blend at a high speed until smooth. (If needed, turn off the blender, stir, and blend again.)

MAKES 1 SERVING

All About Powdered Peanut Butter . . .

Major find here! Powdered peanut butter is made of *defatted* peanuts. How cool is that? The nutritional stats are wildly impressive—a 2-tablespoon serving has about 50 calories and 1.5g fat. Find it at health-food stores and select grocery stores, or order some online. Brand recommendations: FitNutz, PB2, and Just Great Stuff.

PB&J Smoothie

Entire recipe: 325 calories, 8.5g fat, 205mg sodium, 42g carbs, 5.5g fiber, 28g sugars, 21.5g protein

1½ cups frozen unsweetened strawberries, partially thawed

½ cup fat-free milk

½ cup fat-free vanilla Greek yogurt

1 tablespoon powdered peanut butter

1 tablespoon creamy peanut butter

Dash cinnamon

1 no-calorie sweetener packet

1 cup crushed ice *or* 5 to 8 ice cubes

You'll Need: blender

Prep: 5 minutes

Place all ingredients in a blender. Blend at a high speed until smooth. (If needed, turn off the blender, stir, and blend again.)

MAKES 1 SERVING

Berry 'Nana Greens Smoothie

Entire recipe: 318 calories, 5.5g fat, 194mg sodium, 45.5g carbs, 9.5g fiber, 23g sugars, 26g protein

1 cup chopped spinach leaves

1 cup chopped kale leaves

¾ cup fat-free milk

½ cup sliced banana

½ cup frozen unsweetened strawberries, partially thawed

¼ cup vanilla protein powder with about 100 calories per serving

1 tablespoon chia seeds

½ cup crushed ice *or* 3 to 4 ice cubes

You'll Need: blender

Prep: 5 minutes

Place all ingredients in a blender. Blend at high speed until smooth. (If needed, turn off the blender, stir, and blend again.)

MAKES 1 SERVING

> ## HG FYI
> This is one HUGE smoothie!

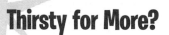

Thirsty for More?

Check out Snack Sips: Smoothies & More! page 271.

Pumped-Up Pancakes, French Toast & Crepes

These aren't your average flapjacks, French toast, and breakfast crepes. These are PUMPED UP with protein. They're also insanely delicious! Try 'em all and see . . .

All About Protein Powder . . .

Never used it before? No worries!

What is it? Protein powder is a shelf-stable source of nutritious protein that can be blended seamlessly into a variety of foods and drinks. The types on shelves run the gamut. They can be made from whey (dairy), soy . . . even brown rice! A couple of my favorite brands are Designer Whey and Quest.

Why use it? Protein powder is a great way to boost the protein count of foods that traditionally wouldn't have a lot of protein: cereal, smoothies, pancakes, and more. And extra protein means they're extra filling.

What else can I do with it? Flip to the index to see all the recipes in this book that call for protein powder. The Protein-Packed Chocolate Cake in a Mug (page 298) is a personal favorite!

PROTEIN POWER!

Pancake Tip!

The first pancake generally takes the longest to cook, so keep an eye on that second one; it'll cook faster!

Strawberry Banana Pancakes

Entire recipe: 320 calories, 6.5g fat, 562mg sodium, 43.5g carbs, 8g fiber, 16.5g sugars, 25g protein

¼ cup egg whites or fat-free liquid egg substitute

¼ cup mashed ripe banana

3 tablespoons vanilla protein powder with about 100 calories per serving

3 tablespoons oat bran

1 no-calorie sweetener packet

½ teaspoon baking powder

⅛ teaspoon vanilla extract

Dash cinnamon

Dash salt

¾ cup sliced strawberries

2 tablespoons fat-free vanilla Greek yogurt

¼ ounce (about 1 tablespoon) sliced almonds

You'll Need: medium bowl, skillet, nonstick spray, plate

Prep: 10 minutes

Cook: 10 minutes

1. To make the batter, in a medium bowl, combine all ingredients *except* strawberries, yogurt, and almonds. Mix until uniform.

2. Bring a skillet sprayed with nonstick spray to medium heat. Add half of the batter to form a large pancake. Cook until it begins to bubble and is solid enough to flip, 1 to 2 minutes.

3. Gently flip, and cook until both sides are lightly browned and inside is cooked through, about 1 minute.

4. Plate your pancake and top with half of the strawberries.

5. Remove skillet from heat, re-spray, and return to medium heat. Repeat with remaining batter to make a second pancake.

6. Place second pancake over the first. Top with remaining strawberries, followed by yogurt and almonds.

MAKES 1 SERVING

Banana Walnut Pancakes 📷

Entire recipe: 319 calories, 7g fat, 556mg sodium, 42g carbs, 6.5g fiber, 15.5g sugars, 24.5g protein

¼ cup egg whites or fat-free liquid egg substitute

¼ cup mashed ripe banana

3 tablespoons vanilla protein powder with about 100 calories per serving

3 tablespoons oat bran

1 no-calorie sweetener packet

½ teaspoon baking powder

⅛ teaspoon vanilla extract

Dash cinnamon

Dash salt

¼ cup sliced banana

2 tablespoons fat-free vanilla Greek yogurt

¼ ounce (about 1 tablespoon) chopped walnuts

You'll Need: medium bowl, skillet, nonstick spray, plate

Prep: 10 minutes

Cook: 10 minutes

1. To make the batter, in a medium bowl, combine all ingredients *except* sliced banana, yogurt, and walnuts. Mix until uniform.

2. Bring a skillet sprayed with nonstick spray to medium heat. Add half of the batter to form a large pancake. Cook until it begins to bubble and is solid enough to flip, 1 to 2 minutes.

3. Gently flip, and cook until both sides are lightly browned and inside is cooked through, about 1 minute.

4. Plate your pancake. Remove skillet from heat, re-spray, and return to medium heat. Repeat with remaining batter to make a second pancake.

5. Plate pancake, and top both with remaining ingredients.

MAKES 1 SERVING

Apple Cinnamon Pancakes

Entire recipe: 318 calories, 6g fat, 568mg sodium, 40.5g carbs, 7g fiber, 18g sugars, 26.5g protein

¼ cup egg whites or fat-free liquid egg substitute

¼ cup no-sugar-added applesauce

3 tablespoons vanilla protein powder with about 100 calories per serving

3 tablespoons oat bran

2 no-calorie sweetener packets

½ teaspoon baking powder

⅛ teaspoon vanilla extract

Dash salt

¼ teaspoon plus 1 dash cinnamon

½ cup finely chopped Fuji apple (or another sweet apple)

¼ cup fat-free vanilla Greek yogurt

¼ ounce (about 1 tablespoon) sliced almonds

You'll Need: medium bowl, small bowl, skillet, nonstick spray, plate

Prep: 10 minutes

Cook: 10 minutes

1. To make the batter, in a medium bowl, combine egg whites/substitute, applesauce, protein powder, oat bran, sweetener, baking powder, vanilla extract, and salt. Add ¼ teaspoon cinnamon and 2 tablespoons water, and mix until smooth and uniform. Stir in apple.

2. In a small bowl, mix remaining dash of cinnamon into yogurt.

3. Bring a skillet sprayed with nonstick spray to medium heat. Add half of the batter to form a large pancake. Cook until it begins to bubble and is solid enough to flip, 1 to 2 minutes.

4. Gently flip, and cook until both sides are lightly browned and inside is cooked through, about 1 minute.

5. Plate your pancake. Remove skillet from heat, re-spray, and return to medium heat. Repeat with remaining batter to make a second pancake.

6. Plate pancake, and top both with yogurt and almonds.

MAKES 1 SERVING

Blueberry Pancakes
with egg scramble

Entire recipe: 328 calories, 5.5g fat, 565mg sodium, 44.5g carbs, 6.5g fiber, 12.5g sugars, 24g protein

PANCAKES

¼ cup whole-wheat flour

2 tablespoons vanilla protein powder with about 100 calories per serving

½ teaspoon baking powder

Dash cinnamon

3 tablespoons egg whites or fat-free liquid egg substitute

¼ cup no-sugar-added applesauce

⅛ teaspoon vanilla extract

1 no-calorie sweetener packet

2½ teaspoons light whipped butter or light buttery spread

½ cup frozen unsweetened blueberries, thawed and drained

¾ teaspoon cornstarch

(continued on next page)

You'll Need: medium bowl, skillet, nonstick spray, plate, medium microwave-safe bowl, microwave-safe mug

Prep: 10 minutes

Cook: 10 minutes

1. To make the pancake batter, in a medium bowl, combine flour, protein powder, baking powder, and cinnamon. Mix well. Add egg whites/substitute, applesauce, and vanilla extract. Add half of the sweetener packet and 2 tablespoons water, and stir until smooth and uniform.

2. Bring a skillet sprayed with nonstick spray to medium heat. Add half of the batter to form a large pancake. Cook until it begins to bubble and is solid enough to flip, 1 to 2 minutes.

3. Gently flip and cook until both sides are lightly browned and inside is cooked through, about 1 minute.

4. Plate the pancake, and spread with 1¼ teaspoons butter. Remove skillet from heat, re-spray, and return to medium heat. Repeat with remaining batter to make a second pancake.

SCRAMBLE

⅓ cup egg whites
or fat-free liquid egg
substitute

Optional seasonings:
garlic powder,
onion powder, black
pepper

5. Place the second pancake over the first, and spread with remaining 1¼ teaspoons butter.

6. Place blueberries in a medium microwave-safe bowl sprayed with nonstick spray. Stir in 1 tablespoon water. Sprinkle with cornstarch, and stir to coat. Microwave for 1 minute, or until hot and thickened. Stir in remaining half of the sweetener packet, and spoon over pancakes.

7. To make the scramble, place egg whites/substitute in a microwave-safe mug sprayed with nonstick spray. Microwave for 45 seconds. Stir and microwave for 15 seconds, or until set. Serve with pancakes.

MAKES 1 SERVING

PB&J French Toast

Entire recipe: 310 calories, 7.5g fat, 410mg sodium, 40.5 carbs, 11g fiber, 13g sugars, 24.5g protein

⅓ cup egg whites or fat-free liquid egg substitute

2 tablespoons vanilla protein powder with about 100 calories per serving

¼ teaspoon cinnamon

¼ teaspoon vanilla extract

1 no-calorie sweetener packet

2 slices light bread

1 cup frozen unsweetened mixed berries, thawed and drained

2 teaspoons creamy peanut butter

You'll Need: wide bowl, whisk, large skillet, nonstick spray, plate, microwave-safe bowl

Prep: 5 minutes

Cook: 5 minutes

1. In a wide bowl, combine egg whites/substitute, protein powder, cinnamon, vanilla extract, and half of the sweetener packet. Whisk thoroughly.

2. Bring a large skillet sprayed with nonstick spray to medium-high heat.

3. Thoroughly soak bread in egg mixture, until all the mixture has been absorbed. Cook until golden brown, 1 to 2 minutes per side. Transfer to a plate.

4. In a microwave-safe bowl, combine berries with peanut butter and the remaining half of the sweetener packet. Microwave for 15 seconds, or until peanut butter is warm. Stir to coat, and spoon over French toast.

MAKES 1 SERVING

Blueberry Almond French Toast

Entire recipe: 322 calories, 9g fat, 425mg sodium, 40g carbs, 9g fiber, 12.5g sugars, 22.5g protein

⅓ cup egg whites or fat-free liquid egg substitute

2 tablespoons vanilla protein powder with about 100 calories per serving

¼ teaspoon cinnamon

¼ teaspoon vanilla extract

2 no-calorie sweetener packets

2 teaspoons light whipped butter or light buttery spread

2 slices light bread

¾ cup frozen unsweetened blueberries, thawed and drained

1 teaspoon cornstarch

¼ ounce (about 1 tablespoon) sliced almonds

You'll Need: wide bowl, whisk, large skillet, nonstick spray, plate, microwave-safe bowl

Prep: 5 minutes

Cook: 5 minutes

1. In a wide bowl, combine egg whites/substitute, protein powder, cinnamon, vanilla extract, and 1 sweetener packet. Whisk thoroughly.

2. Bring a large skillet sprayed with nonstick spray to medium-high heat. Add butter, and let it coat the bottom.

3. Thoroughly soak bread in egg mixture, until all the mixture has been absorbed. Cook until golden brown, 1 to 2 minutes per side. Transfer to a plate.

4. Place berries in a microwave-safe bowl sprayed with nonstick spray. Stir in 1½ tablespoons water. Sprinkle with cornstarch, and stir to coat. Microwave for 1 minute, or until hot and thickened. Stir in remaining sweetener packet, and spoon over French toast. Top with almonds.

MAKES 1 SERVING

Stuffed 'n Smothered Berry French Toast 📷

Entire recipe: 323 calories, 8.5g fat, 482mg sodium, 43.5g carbs, 9g fiber, 16.5g sugars, 20.5g protein

¼ cup egg whites or fat-free liquid egg substitute

¼ teaspoon vanilla extract

¼ teaspoon cinnamon

⅓ cup light/low-fat ricotta cheese

1 no-calorie sweetener packet

2 teaspoons light whipped butter or light buttery spread

2 slices light bread

½ cup sliced strawberries

½ cup frozen unsweetened blueberries, thawed and drained

1½ teaspoons cornstarch

You'll Need: wide bowl, whisk, small bowl, large skillet, nonstick spray, plate, medium microwave-safe bowl

Prep: 5 minutes

Cook: 5 minutes

1. In a wide bowl, combine egg whites/substitute, ⅛ teaspoon vanilla extract, and ⅛ teaspoon cinnamon. Whisk thoroughly.

2. In a small bowl, combine ricotta cheese, half of the sweetener packet, remaining ⅛ teaspoon vanilla extract, and remaining ⅛ teaspoon cinnamon. Mix well.

3. Bring a large skillet sprayed with nonstick spray to medium-high heat. Add butter, and let it coat the bottom.

4. Thoroughly soak bread in egg mixture, until all the mixture has been absorbed. Cook until golden brown, 1 to 2 minutes per side. Transfer to a plate.

5. Spread ricotta mixture onto one slice of French toast. Top with the other piece of French toast, and lightly press to seal. Top with strawberries.

6. Place blueberries in a medium microwave-safe bowl sprayed with nonstick spray. Stir in 1½ tablespoons water. Sprinkle with cornstarch, and stir to coat. Microwave for 1 minute, or until hot and thickened. Stir in remaining half of the sweetener packet, and spoon over French toast.

MAKES 1 SERVING

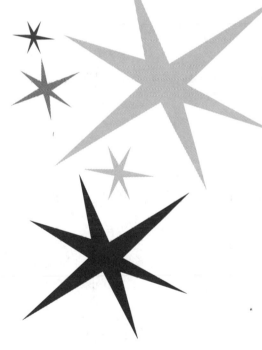

Peaches & Cream Stuffed French Toast

Entire recipe: 318 calories, 8g fat, 480mg sodium, 43g carbs, 8g fiber, 19.5g sugars, 21g protein

¼ cup egg whites or fat-free liquid egg substitute

¼ teaspoon vanilla extract

¼ teaspoon cinnamon

⅓ cup light/low-fat ricotta cheese

1 no-calorie sweetener packet

2 teaspoons light whipped butter or light buttery spread

2 slices light bread

1 cup chopped peaches (fresh or thawed from frozen)

1½ teaspoons cornstarch

You'll Need: wide bowl, whisk, small bowl, large skillet, nonstick spray, plate, medium microwave-safe bowl

Prep: 5 minutes

Cook: 10 minutes

1. In a wide bowl, combine egg whites/substitute, ⅛ teaspoon vanilla extract, and ⅛ teaspoon cinnamon. Whisk thoroughly.

2. In a small bowl, combine ricotta cheese, half of the sweetener packet, remaining ⅛ teaspoon vanilla extract, and remaining ⅛ teaspoon cinnamon. Mix well.

3. Bring a large skillet sprayed with nonstick spray to medium-high heat. Add butter, and let it coat the bottom.

4. Thoroughly soak bread in egg mixture, until all the mixture has been absorbed. Cook until golden brown, 1 to 2 minutes per side. Transfer to a plate.

5. Spread ricotta mixture onto one slice of French toast. Top with the other piece of French toast, and lightly press to seal.

6. Place peaches in a medium microwave-safe bowl sprayed with nonstick spray. Stir in 1½ tablespoons water. Sprinkle with cornstarch, and stir to coat. Microwave for 1½ minutes, or until hot and thickened. Stir in remaining half of the sweetener packet, and spoon over French toast.

MAKES 1 SERVING

All About HG-Style Crepes . . .

The crepes in this book are super-thin pancakes made from egg whites and protein powder—they're basically PURE PROTEIN. They sound fancy, but they're extremely easy to make. Here are some things to keep in mind . . .

- A 10-inch skillet is essential. Any smaller, and your crepe will be too thick; any larger, and your crepe will be too thin. (Yes, there *is* such a thing as being too thin . . . especially if you're a crepe!)

- That offset spatula the recipes call for? It's just a flipping utensil with a handy bend in the blade, which allows you to gently get underneath the crepe without breaking it.

- When you're mixing up the batter, don't stress if it isn't completely uniform. Any bits of protein powder will break up while the batter cooks.

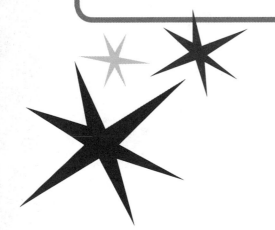

Strawberry Almond Crepes

Entire recipe: 330 calories, 8.5g fat, 262mg sodium, 40g carbs, 6.5g fiber, 28g sugars, 26g protein

½ cup egg whites

2 tablespoons vanilla protein powder with about 100 calories per serving

⅛ teaspoon vanilla extract

⅛ teaspoon cinnamon

¼ cup fat-free vanilla yogurt

2 tablespoons low-sugar strawberry preserves

1¼ cups sliced strawberries

½ ounce (about 2 tablespoons) sliced almonds

You'll Need: small bowl, whisk, 10-inch skillet, nonstick spray, offset spatula or flexible rubber spatula, plate, medium bowl

Prep: 5 minutes

Cook: 10 minutes

1. To make the batter, in a small bowl, combine egg whites, protein powder, vanilla extract, and cinnamon. Whisk until uniform.

2. To make the crepes, bring a 10-inch skillet sprayed with nonstick spray to medium heat. Pour half of the batter into the pan, quickly tilting the skillet in all directions to evenly coat the bottom. Cook until lightly browned on the bottom, about 2 minutes. Carefully flip with an offset spatula or flexible rubber spatula. Cook until lightly browned on the other side, about 1 minute.

3. Transfer the crepe to a plate, and repeat with remaining egg mixture to make another crepe.

4. In a medium bowl, mix yogurt with preserves until uniform. Add strawberries and almonds, and stir to coat. Divide mixture between the centers of the crepes.

5. Fold both sides of each crepe over the filling.

MAKES 1 SERVING

Apple Strudel Crepes 📷

Entire recipe: 330 calories, 6.5g fat, 247mg sodium, 40.5g carbs, 5g fiber, 21g sugars, 28g protein

¼ cup old-fashioned oats

1 no-calorie sweetener packet

½ cup egg whites

1½ tablespoons vanilla protein powder with about 100 calories per serving

¼ teaspoon cinnamon

⅛ teaspoon vanilla extract

½ cup finely chopped apple

¼ cup fat-free plain Greek yogurt

1½ tablespoons raisins

¼ ounce (about 1 tablespoon) chopped walnuts

You'll Need: medium-large microwave-safe bowl, small bowl, whisk, 10-inch skillet, nonstick spray, offset spatula or flexible rubber spatula, plate

Prep: 5 minutes

Cook: 10 minutes

1. In a medium-large microwave-safe bowl, mix oats with ½ cup water. Microwave for 2 minutes, or until thickened. Add sweetener, and stir well.

2. To make the batter, in a small bowl, combine egg whites, protein powder, cinnamon, and vanilla extract. Whisk until uniform.

3. To make the crepes, bring a 10-inch skillet sprayed with nonstick spray to medium heat. Pour half of the batter into the pan, quickly tilting the skillet in all directions to evenly coat the bottom. Cook until lightly browned on the bottom, about 2 minutes. Carefully flip with an offset spatula or flexible rubber spatula. Cook until lightly browned on the other side, about 1 minute.

4. Transfer the crepe to a plate, and repeat with remaining egg mixture to make another crepe.

5. To the bowl of cooked oats, add apple, yogurt, raisins, and walnuts. Mix well. Divide mixture between the centers of the crepes.

6. Fold both sides of each crepe over the filling.

MAKES 1 SERVING

Chocolate Raspberry Coconut Crepes

Entire recipe; 327 calories, 8.5g fat, 291mg sodium, 39g carbs, 11.5g fiber, 25g sugars, 24g protein

½ cup egg whites

2 tablespoons chocolate protein powder with about 100 calories per serving

⅛ teaspoon vanilla extract

⅛ teaspoon cinnamon

¼ cup fat-free vanilla yogurt

1½ tablespoons shredded sweetened coconut

1 tablespoon mini semi-sweet chocolate chips

1 cup raspberries

You'll Need: small bowl, whisk, 10-inch skillet, nonstick spray, offset spatula or flexible rubber spatula, plate, medium bowl

Prep: 5 minutes

Cook: 10 minutes

1. To make the batter, in a small bowl, combine egg whites, protein powder, vanilla extract, and cinnamon. Whisk until uniform.

2. To make the crepes, bring a 10-inch skillet sprayed with nonstick spray to medium heat. Pour half of the batter into the pan, quickly tilting the skillet in all directions to evenly coat the bottom. Cook until lightly browned on the bottom, about 2 minutes. Carefully flip with an offset spatula or flexible rubber spatula. Cook until lightly browned on the other side, about 1 minute.

3. Transfer the crepe to a plate, and repeat with remaining egg mixture to make another crepe.

4. In a medium bowl, combine yogurt, coconut, and chocolate chips. Mix well. Gently stir in raspberries. Divide mixture between the centers of the crepes.

5. Fold both sides of each crepe over the filling.

MAKES 1 SERVING

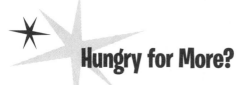

Hungry for More?

Don't miss the Breakfast-Style Burrito Crepes (page 124) and the Lemon Blueberry Crepe (page 290)!

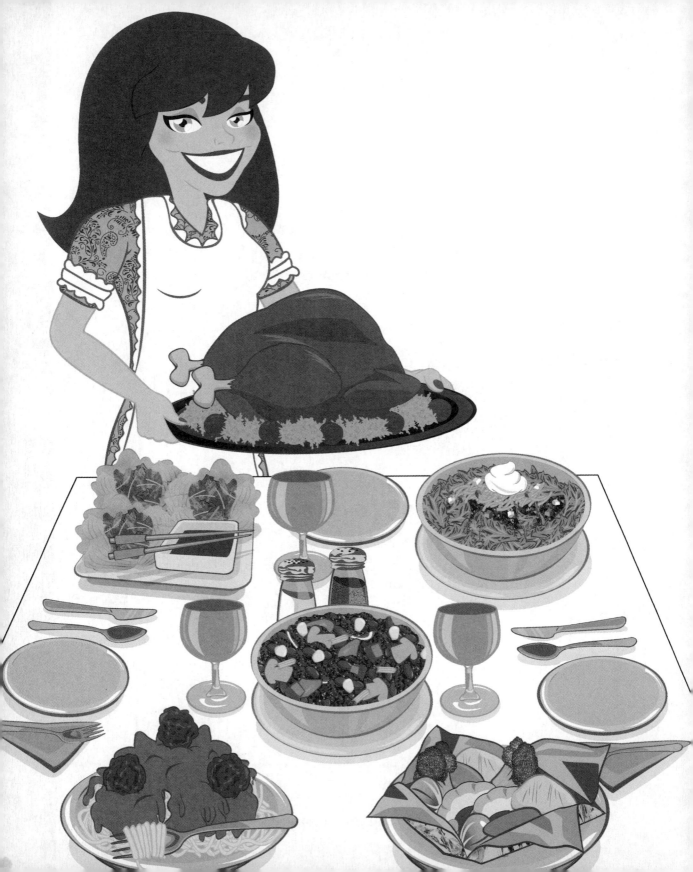

LUNCHES & DINNERS

Stir-Frys, Skillets & Grills

These stovetop entrées are easy and incredible. Perfect for a weeknight dinner or a make-ahead lunch. So much good stuff here!

Chinese Chicken Stir-Fry 📷

Entire recipe: 350 calories, 7g fat, 730mg sodium, 33.5g carbs, 7g fiber, 20g sugars, 32.5g protein

SAUCE

2½ teaspoons reduced-sodium/lite soy sauce

1½ teaspoons brown sugar (not packed)

1 teaspoon Asian-style chili garlic sauce

¼ teaspoon sesame oil or olive oil

STIR-FRY

2½ cups frozen Asian-style stir-fry vegetables

4 ounces raw boneless skinless chicken breast, cut into bite-sized pieces

⅛ teaspoon garlic powder

⅛ teaspoon black pepper

2 tablespoons canned sliced water chestnuts, drained and roughly chopped

¼ cup mandarin orange segments packed in juice, drained

2 tablespoons chopped scallions

¼ ounce (about 1 tablespoon) sliced almonds

You'll Need: small bowl, skillet, nonstick spray

Prep: 10 minutes

Cook: 15 minutes

1. In a small bowl, combine sauce ingredients with 1 tablespoon water. Mix thoroughly.

2. Bring a skillet sprayed with nonstick spray to medium-high heat. Cook and stir frozen veggies until thawed, 4 to 6 minutes.

3. Add chicken to the skillet, and season with garlic powder and pepper. Cook and stir until veggies are hot and chicken is fully cooked, about 4 minutes.

4. Remove skillet from heat. Stir sauce mixture, and add to the skillet, along with water chestnuts. Mix well.

5. Serve topped with orange segments, scallions, and almonds.

MAKES 1 SERVING

Beef Teriyaki Stir-Fry

Entire recipe: 334 calories, 7.5g fat, 655mg sodium, 32g carbs, 9g fiber, 10.5g sugars, 35.5g protein

3 cups small broccoli florets

1 cup halved sugar snap peas

4 ounces thinly sliced raw lean beefsteak

Dash garlic powder

Dash onion powder

¼ cup canned sliced water chestnuts, drained and roughly chopped

2 tablespoons teriyaki sauce or marinade with 25 calories or less per tablespoon

You'll Need: large skillet, nonstick spray

Prep: 10 minutes

Cook: 10 minutes

1. Bring a large skillet sprayed with nonstick spray to medium-high heat. Add broccoli, sugar snap peas, and ¼ cup water. Cook and stir until water has evaporated and veggies have slightly softened, about 3 minutes.

2. Add beef to the skillet, and season with garlic powder and onion powder. Cook and stir until veggies have softened and beef is cooked through, about 2 minutes.

3. Remove from heat, and add water chestnuts and sauce/marinade. Mix well.

MAKES 1 SERVING

HG Tip!

Freeze your beef fillet slightly before cutting into it; this will make it easier to slice.

Stir-Frys, Skillets & Grills

Southwestern Stir-Fry

Entire recipe: 347 calories, 8g fat, 458mg sodium, 37.5g carbs, 10g fiber, 10.5g sugars, 36g protein

4 ounces raw extra-lean ground beef (4% fat or less)

¼ cup chopped onion

1 teaspoon taco seasoning mix

2 cups small broccoli florets

1 portabella mushroom, sliced

3 tablespoons frozen sweet corn kernels

3 tablespoons canned black beans, drained and rinsed

1 tablespoon light sour cream

Optional seasoning: salt-free seasoning mix (Southwestern variety, if available)

You'll Need: skillet, nonstick spray, small bowl

Prep: 10 minutes

Cook: 10 minutes

1. Bring a skillet sprayed with nonstick spray to medium-high heat. Add beef and onion. Cook, stir, and crumble until beef is fully cooked and onion has softened and lightly browned, about 4 minutes. Add ½ teaspoon taco seasoning, and stir until well mixed.

2. Transfer beef mixture to a small bowl, and cover to keep warm.

3. Remove skillet from heat; clean, if needed. Re-spray, and return to medium-high heat. Add broccoli, mushroom, corn, and 2 tablespoons water. Cook and stir until water has evaporated and veggies have softened, about 4 minutes.

4. Return beef mixture to the skillet. Add beans, sour cream, and remaining ½ teaspoon taco seasoning. Cook and stir until hot and well mixed, about 1 minute.

MAKES 1 SERVING

Saucy Mexican Stir-Fry

Entire recipe: 336 calories, 7g fat, 658mg sodium, 34.5g carbs, 14g fiber, 11g sugars, 34g protein

3 cups bagged broccoli cole slaw

4 ounces raw extra-lean ground beef (4% fat or less)

1 teaspoon taco seasoning mix

2 tablespoons frozen sweet corn kernels

½ cup canned crushed tomatoes

2 tablespoons canned black beans, drained and rinsed

Dash ground cumin

Dash chili powder

½ ounce (about 1 tablespoon) chopped avocado

You'll Need: large skillet with a lid, nonstick spray, medium bowl

Prep: 5 minutes

Cook: 20 minutes

1. Bring a large skillet sprayed with nonstick spray to medium-high heat. Add broccoli slaw and ½ cup water. Cover and cook for 8 minutes, or until fully softened. Uncover and, if needed, cook and stir until water has evaporated, 1 to 2 minutes. Transfer to a medium bowl, and cover to keep warm.

2. Remove skillet from heat, re-spray, and return to medium-high heat. Add beef, and sprinkle with ½ teaspoon taco seasoning. Cook and crumble until fully cooked, 2 to 3 minutes. Transfer to the bowl, and re-cover to keep warm.

3. Remove skillet from heat; clean, if needed. Re-spray, and return to medium-high heat. Cook and stir corn until hot and slightly blackened, 1 to 2 minutes.

4. Reduce heat to medium. Add contents of the bowl and remaining ½ teaspoon taco seasoning. Add crushed tomatoes, beans, cumin, and chili powder. Cook and stir until hot and well mixed, about 2 minutes.

5. Serve topped with avocado.

MAKES 1 SERVING

Stir-Frys, Skillets & Grills 93

Sweet 'n Spicy Shrimp Stir-Fry 📷

Entire recipe: 342 calories, 8.5g fat, 717mg sodium, 34.5g carbs, 6g fiber, 18g sugars, 31.5g protein

½ cup sliced onion

1 cup bean sprouts

½ cup sugar snap peas

½ cup carrot thinly sliced into coins

1½ teaspoons sesame oil or olive oil

5 ounces (about 9) raw large shrimp, peeled, tails removed, deveined

¼ cup canned sliced water chestnuts, drained and roughly chopped

1 tablespoon sweet Asian chili sauce

⅛ teaspoon red pepper flakes

You'll Need: skillet, nonstick spray

Prep: 10 minutes

Cook: 10 minutes

1. Bring a skillet sprayed with nonstick spray to medium-high heat. Add onion, bean sprouts, snap peas, and carrot. Drizzle with oil, and cook and stir until mostly softened, about 5 minutes.

2. Add shrimp and water chestnuts. Cook and stir until veggies have softened and shrimp are cooked through, about 3 minutes.

3. Remove skillet from heat, and mix in chili sauce and red pepper flakes.

MAKES 1 SERVING

📷 Photo Alert!

The camera icon next to the recipe name means flip to the insert to see a photo of this recipe. Find full-color photos of ALL the recipes at hungry-girl.com/books.

Salmon 'n Snow Pea Stir-Fry

Entire recipe: 350 calories, 11g fat, 613mg sodium, 33g carbs, 8g fiber, 17.5g sugars, 28.5g protein

1½ cups sliced bell pepper

1½ cups snow peas

½ cup sliced onion

½ cup carrot sliced into coins

2 tablespoons teriyaki sauce or marinade with 25 calories or less per 1-tablespoon serving

4 ounces raw skinless salmon, cut into 1-inch cubes

¼ teaspoon salt-free seasoning mix

You'll Need: large skillet, nonstick spray, medium-large bowl

Prep: 10 minutes

Cook: 15 minutes

1. Bring a large skillet sprayed with nonstick spray to medium-high heat. Add pepper, snow peas, onion, carrot, and 2 tablespoons water. Cook and stir until water has evaporated and veggies have mostly softened and slightly browned, about 5 minutes.

2. Add sauce/marinade, and cook and stir until hot and well mixed, about 1 minute. Transfer to a medium-large bowl, and cover to keep warm.

3. Remove skillet from heat; clean, if needed. Re-spray, and return to medium-high heat. Add salmon, and sprinkle with salt-free seasoning. Cook for about 4 minutes, until cooked through, gently flipping to cook on all sides. Top veggies with salmon.

MAKES 1 SERVING

Chicken-Pounding 101

It's as easy as 1-2 . . .

1. Either lay the cutlet between two pieces of plastic wrap or place it in a sealable bag and squeeze out the air before sealing.

2. Starting with the thickest point, pound the cutlet with a meat mallet until it's the desired thickness. Don't have a mallet? Any heavy kitchen tool with a flat surface will do.

Chicken Skillet 'n Cheesy Mashies

Entire recipe: 330 calories, 6.5g fat, 665mg sodium, 29g carbs, 11.5g fiber, 14g sugars, 40g protein

2 cups frozen cauliflower florets

1 tablespoon grated Parmesan cheese

1 wedge The Laughing Cow Light Creamy Swiss cheese

Dash garlic powder

Dash onion powder

Dash each salt and black pepper

One 4-ounce raw boneless skinless chicken breast cutlet, pounded to ½-inch thickness

2 cups sugar snap peas, red bell pepper, carrots, and/or other high-fiber veggies (page 345)

1 teaspoon salt-free seasoning mix

You'll Need: large microwave-safe bowl, skillet, nonstick spray

Prep: 10 minutes

Cook: 20 minutes

1. Place cauliflower in a large microwave-safe bowl. Add 2 tablespoons water, cover, and microwave for 3 minutes.

2. Uncover and stir. Re-cover and microwave for 2 minutes, or until soft.

3. Drain excess liquid. Add Parmesan cheese and cheese wedge, breaking the wedge into pieces. Add garlic powder, onion powder, salt, and pepper. Thoroughly mash and mix. Cover to keep warm.

4. Bring a skillet sprayed with nonstick spray to medium heat. Cook chicken for 5 minutes.

5. Flip chicken, and add veggies to the skillet. Stirring veggies occasionally, cook for about 6 minutes, until chicken is cooked through and veggies have mostly softened.

6. Sprinkle chicken and veggies with salt-free seasoning. If needed, reheat cauliflower mashies.

MAKES 1 SERVING

Mango Avocado Chicken Skillet
with steamed veggies 📷

Entire recipe: 340 calories, 8g fat, 240mg sodium, 36.5g carbs, 6.5g fiber, 24g sugars, 32g protein

1½ tablespoons balsamic vinegar

½ tablespoon honey

One 4.5-ounce raw boneless skinless chicken breast cutlet, pounded to ½-inch thickness

¼ teaspoon garlic powder

¼ teaspoon onion powder

Dash each salt and black pepper

1 cup sugar snap peas, red bell pepper, carrots, and/ or other high-fiber veggies (page 345)

¼ teaspoon salt-free seasoning mix

½ cup sliced onion

¼ cup chopped mango

½ teaspoon chopped garlic

1 ounce (about 2 tablespoons) chopped avocado

You'll Need: small bowl, large sealable bag, medium microwave-safe bowl, large skillet, nonstick spray

Prep: 10 minutes

Marinate: 30 minutes

Cook: 15 minutes

1. In a small bowl, combine vinegar, honey, and 1 tablespoon water. Mix until uniform. Transfer to a large sealable bag.

2. Season chicken with garlic powder, onion powder, salt, and pepper. Add to the bag and seal, removing as much air as possible. Marinate in the fridge for 30 minutes.

3. In a medium microwave-safe bowl, combine veggies with 2 tablespoons water. Microwave for 3 minutes, or until softened. Drain excess water, and sprinkle with salt-free seasoning. Re-cover to keep warm.

4. Bring a large skillet sprayed with nonstick spray to medium heat. Add chicken, and discard excess marinade. Cook for 5 minutes.

5. Flip chicken. Add onion. Stirring onion occasionally, cook for about 5 more minutes, until chicken is cooked through and blackened and onion has softened.

6. Add mango and garlic, and cook and stir until hot and fragrant, about 1 minute.

7. Serve topped with avocado and alongside steamed veggies.

MAKES 1 SERVING

For the latest food news, recipes, tips 'n tricks, and more, **sign up for free daily emails at hungry-girl.com!**

Big Beef Skillet

½ of recipe (about 2 cups): 334 calories, 7.5g fat, 719mg sodium, 30g carbs, 6g fiber, 12g sugars, 36.5g protein

3 cups bagged cole slaw mix

1⅓ cups chopped green bell pepper

¾ cup fat-free or nearly fat-free beef or turkey gravy

3 cups chopped brown mushrooms

1¼ cups chopped onion

10 ounces raw extra-lean ground beef (4% fat or less)

2 teaspoons onion soup/dip seasoning mix

You'll Need: large skillet, nonstick spray, large bowl

Prep: 15 minutes

Cook: 20 minutes

1. Bring a large skillet sprayed with nonstick spray to medium-high heat. Add cole slaw mix, pepper, and ½ cup water. Cover and cook for 8 minutes, or until fully softened. Uncover and, if needed, cook and stir until water has evaporated, about 1 minute.

2. Add gravy, and cook and stir until hot, about 1 minute. Transfer to a large bowl, and cover to keep warm.

3. Remove skillet from heat; clean, if needed. Re-spray, and return to medium-high heat. Add mushrooms and onion. Cook and stir until slightly softened, about 3 minutes. Add beef, and sprinkle with onion seasoning mix. Cook and crumble until veggies are soft and beef is fully cooked, about 6 minutes.

4. Transfer mixture to the large bowl. Mix well.

MAKES 2 SERVINGS

Upside-Down Shepherd's Pie

¼ of recipe (about 2¼ cups): 350 calories, 9g fat, 689mg sodium, 34g carbs, 10.5g fiber, 12.5g sugars, 33.5g protein

10 cups frozen cauliflower florets

1 cup chopped mushrooms

½ cup chopped onion

1 pound raw extra-lean ground beef (4% fat or less)

1 teaspoon chopped garlic

4 cups frozen petite mixed vegetables, thawed and drained

1 cup fat-free or nearly fat-free beef or turkey gravy

¾ teaspoon garlic powder

¾ teaspoon onion powder

2½ tablespoons light whipped butter or light buttery spread

¼ teaspoon each salt and pepper

HG Tip!

For extra-creamy mashies, blend them in a blender or food processor until smooth.

You'll Need: large microwave-safe bowl, large skillet, nonstick spray

Prep: 10 minutes

Cook: 20 minutes

1. Place cauliflower in a large microwave-safe bowl. Add ¼ cup water, cover, and microwave for 8 minutes. Uncover and stir. Re-cover and microwave for 8 minutes, or until soft.

2. Meanwhile, bring a large skillet sprayed with nonstick spray to medium-high heat. Add mushrooms and onion. Cook and stir until slightly softened, about 2 minutes. Add beef and chopped garlic. Cook and crumble until veggies are soft and beef is fully cooked, about 6 minutes.

3. To the skillet, add thawed veggies, gravy, and ¼ teaspoon each garlic powder and onion powder. Cook and stir until hot, about 5 minutes.

4. Drain excess liquid from cauliflower. Add butter, salt, pepper, and remaining ½ teaspoon each garlic powder and onion powder. Thoroughly mash and mix.

5. Top each serving of the cauliflower mixture (about 1 cup) with a serving of the beef mixture (about 1¼ cups).

MAKES 4 SERVINGS

Stir-Frys, Skillets & Grills   **101**

Unstuffed Cabbage Rolls
with side salad

Entire recipe: 349 calories, 9g fat, 465mg sodium, 32.5g carbs, 9.5g fiber, 18g sugars, 36.5g protein

CABBAGE ROLLS

5 ounces raw extra-lean ground beef (4% fat or less)

¼ cup chopped onion

¼ teaspoon onion powder

¼ teaspoon garlic powder

2 cups roughly chopped cabbage

½ cup chopped tomato

¼ cup canned crushed tomatoes

1 teaspoon chopped garlic

⅛ teaspoon black pepper

Dash salt

½ teaspoon cider vinegar

(continued on next page)

You'll Need: skillet with a lid, nonstick spray, medium bowl

Prep: 10 minutes

Cook: 15 minutes

1. Bring a skillet sprayed with nonstick spray to medium-high heat. Add beef, onion, and ⅛ teaspoon each onion powder and garlic powder. Cook, stir, and crumble until beef is fully cooked and onion has softened and lightly browned, 4 to 5 minutes.

2. Reduce heat to medium low. Add cabbage, chopped tomato, crushed tomatoes, chopped garlic, pepper, and salt. Add 1 tablespoon water and remaining ⅛ teaspoon each onion powder and garlic powder. Mix well.

3. Cover and cook for 10 minutes, or until cabbage is tender.

SIDE SALAD

1 cup lettuce

½ cup tomatoes, onions, and/or other high-fiber veggies (page 345)

½ cup cucumber, mushrooms, and/or other high-volume veggies (page 345)

2½ teaspoons balsamic, red wine, or white wine vinegar

½ teaspoon extra-virgin olive oil or grapeseed oil

4. Meanwhile, toss salad ingredients in a medium bowl.

5. Stir cider vinegar into cabbage mixture, and serve with salad.

MAKES 1 SERVING

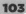

Chicken Marinara Stuffed Potato 📷

Entire recipe: 338 calories, 7g fat, 707mg sodium, 31.5g carbs, 4.5g fiber, 5.5g sugars, 37g protein

One 10-ounce russet potato

4½ ounces raw boneless skinless chicken breast, cut into bite-sized pieces

⅛ teaspoon each salt and black pepper

¼ cup chopped mushrooms

2 tablespoons chopped onion

¼ cup low-fat marinara sauce

¼ teaspoon garlic powder

1 tablespoon grated Parmesan cheese

You'll Need: microwave-safe plate, skillet, nonstick spray

Prep: 10 minutes

Cook: 15 minutes

1. Pierce potato several times with a fork. On a microwave-safe plate, microwave potato for 3½ minutes.

2. Flip potato, and microwave for another 3½ minutes, or until soft.

3. Once cool enough to handle, cut potato in half lengthwise. Use a spoon to gently scoop out the pulp, leaving about ¼ inch inside the skin. Discard the potato pulp (or reserve for another use).

4. Bring a skillet sprayed with nonstick spray to medium-high heat. Add chicken, and sprinkle with salt and pepper. Add mushrooms and onion, and cook and stir for about 4 minutes, until chicken is fully cooked and veggies have softened and browned.

5. Remove skillet from heat. Add marinara sauce, garlic powder, and 1½ teaspoons Parm. Stir to coat. Divide mixture between the potato halves.

6. Sprinkle with remaining 1½ teaspoons Parm.

MAKES 1 SERVING

Butternut Squash & Chicken Sausage Skillet 📷

½ of recipe (2¼ cups): 337 calories, 8.5g fat, 665mg sodium, 38g carbs, 6.5g fiber, 11g sugars, 31g protein

3 cups cubed butternut squash

2 cups sliced mushrooms

½ cup chopped apple

½ cup chopped onion

¼ teaspoon dried ground sage

⅛ teaspoon black pepper

Dash salt

6 ounces (about 2 links) fully cooked chicken sausage with 8g fat or less per 3-ounce serving, sliced into coins

3 ounces cooked and chopped skinless chicken breast

1 teaspoon chopped garlic

You'll Need: large skillet with a lid, nonstick spray

Prep: 20 minutes

Cook: 15 minutes

1. Bring a large skillet sprayed with nonstick spray to medium heat. Add squash and ½ cup water. Cover and cook until water has evaporated and squash has mostly softened, about 8 minutes, uncovering occasionally to stir.

2. Raise heat to medium high. Add mushrooms, apple, onion, sage, pepper, and salt. Cook and stir until veggies have softened and excess liquid has evaporated, about 3 minutes.

3. Add sausage coins, chicken, and garlic. Cook and stir until hot, about 3 more minutes.

MAKES 2 SERVINGS

Need Chicken Cooking Tips?

Check out page 319, or purchase precooked chicken!

Chicken & Romaine Grill
with steamed veggies

Entire recipe: 341 calories, 10.5g fat, 596mg sodium, 29g carbs, 9g fiber, 15g sugars, 33.5g protein

Half of a large heart romaine lettuce (halved lengthwise)

1 teaspoon olive oil or grapeseed oil

Dash each salt and black pepper

2 tablespoons diced tomato

2 tablespoons diced red onion

1 tablespoon crumbled reduced-fat feta cheese

One 4-ounce raw boneless skinless chicken breast cutlet, pounded to ½-inch thickness

1½ cups sugar snap peas, red bell pepper, carrots, and/or other high-fiber veggies (page 345)

1 cup zucchini, cauliflower, and/or other high-volume veggies (page 345)

(continued on next page)

You'll Need: grill pan, nonstick spray, plate, large microwave-safe bowl, small bowl, whisk

Prep: 15 minutes

Cook: 10 minutes

1. Bring a grill pan sprayed with nonstick spray to high heat.

2. Drizzle ½ teaspoon oil onto the cut sides of the romaine half. Sprinkle with salt and black pepper. Grill until slightly charred, 1 to 2 minutes.

3. Plate romaine half, cut side up. Top with tomato, onion, and feta cheese.

4. Remove grill pan from heat; clean, if needed. Respray, and bring to medium heat. Grill chicken until cooked through, about 3 minutes per side.

5. Meanwhile, place remaining veggies in a large microwave-safe bowl. Add 2 tablespoons water, cover, and microwave for 3 minutes, or until softened.

1 tablespoon sauce, dressing, or marinade with 25 calories or less per 1-tablespoon serving

½ teaspoon salt-free seasoning mix

1 tablespoon balsamic vinegar

6. Drain excess water from veggies. Drizzle with 1½ teaspoons sauce/dressing/marinade.

7. Sprinkle cooked chicken with salt-free seasoning, and drizzle with remaining 1½ teaspoons sauce/ dressing/marinade.

8. In a small bowl, whisk vinegar with remaining ½ teaspoon oil. Drizzle over grilled romaine.

MAKES 1 SERVING

No Grill Pan? No Problem!

While grill marks are *awesome* and grilled food tastes fantastic, when our recipes call for a grill pan, you can use a large skillet instead. But seriously consider adding a grill pan to your cooking collection!

Chicken & Veggie Kebabs

Entire recipe: 340 calories, 10.5g fat, 681mg sodium, 23g carbs, 4g fiber, 13.5g sugars, 36.5g protein

2½ tablespoons sauce, dressing, or marinade with 25 calories or less per 1-tablespoon serving

1 teaspoon olive oil or grapeseed oil

5 ounces raw boneless skinless chicken breast, cut into 1-inch cubes

1 small zucchini, stem removed, cut into 1-inch pieces

Half of a red bell pepper, stem and seeds removed, cut into 1-inch pieces

½ cup onion cut into 1-inch chunks

6 small mushrooms (about 1-inch wide)

You'll Need: 3 skewers, small bowl, large sealable bag, grill pan, nonstick spray

Prep: 15 minutes

Marinate: 30 minutes

Cook: 15 minutes

1. In a small bowl, mix sauce/dressing/marinade with oil. Place mixture in a large sealable bag. Add all remaining ingredients. Seal bag, removing as much air as possible. Gently knead marinade mixture into chicken and veggies through the bag. Refrigerate for 30 minutes.

2. Alternately thread chicken and veggies onto three skewers. (Discard excess marinade.)

3. Bring a grill pan sprayed with nonstick spray to medium-high heat. Cook kebabs for 5 minutes.

4. Flip kebabs. Cook for 6 to 8 minutes, until chicken is cooked through.

MAKES 1 SERVING

HG Tip!

If using wooden skewers, soak them in water for 20 minutes to prevent burning.

Grilly Island Burger Stack

Entire recipe: 339 calories, 9.5g fat, 696mg sodium, 31.5g carbs, 10g fiber, 12g sugars, 33g protein

2 frozen meatless hamburger-style patties with 100 calories or less each

1 slice pineapple

One ¼-inch-thick slice onion, rings intact

Half of a red bell pepper, stem and seeds removed, cut into strips

1 slice Sargento Reduced Fat Swiss cheese

2 tablespoons fat-free plain Greek yogurt

1 teaspoon balsamic vinegar

Optional seasoning: cayenne pepper

You'll Need: grill pan, nonstick spray, small bowl, plate

Prep: 10 minutes

Cook: 10 minutes

1. Bring a grill pan sprayed with nonstick spray to medium heat. Lay burger patties, pineapple, onion, and pepper strips in the pan. Cook for 5 minutes.

2. Flip contents of the pan. Top one burger patty with cheese. Cook for about 5 more minutes, until burger patties are cooked through and fruit/veggies have softened and lightly browned.

3. Meanwhile, in a small bowl, mix yogurt with vinegar until uniform.

4. To assemble, layer ingredients on a plate in the following order: plain burger patty, half of the pepper strips, half of the yogurt mixture, onion, remaining pepper strips, remaining yogurt mixture, cheese-topped burger patty, and pineapple.

MAKES 1 SERVING

Balsamic Tofu 'n Veggie Grill
with side salad

Entire recipe: 330 calories, 9.5g fat, 645mg sodium, 35.5g carbs, 9.5g fiber, 19.5g sugars, 30g protein

TOFU AND VEGGIES

1½ tablespoons balsamic vinegar

Half of a small red bell pepper (cut lengthwise), stem and seeds removed

1 small zucchini, ends removed

1 portabella mushroom cap (stem removed)

4 ounces block-style extra-firm tofu, cut into 2 slices about ½-inch thick

2 large tomato slices

2 dashes salt

¼ teaspoon garlic powder

¼ teaspoon onion powder

⅛ teaspoon black pepper

(continued on next page)

You'll Need: wide bowl, grill pan, nonstick spray, plate, medium bowl

Prep: 15 minutes

Cook: 15 minutes

1. Place balsamic vinegar in a wide bowl.

2. Cut bell pepper half lengthwise into two pieces, and cut the zucchini lengthwise into two pieces.

3. Spray a grill pan with nonstick spray, and bring to medium-high heat.

4. One at a time, coat bell pepper pieces, zucchini pieces, and portabella mushroom cap with balsamic vinegar, and lay them on the grill pan. Grill until softened and slightly blackened, about 5 minutes per side.

5. Plate grilled veggies. Remove grill pan from heat; clean, if needed. Re-spray, and return to medium-high heat.

6. Coat tofu slices with balsamic vinegar. Lay tofu and tomato on the grill pan, and sprinkle tofu with salt. Grill until slightly blackened, about 2 minutes per side.

SIDE SALAD

2 cups lettuce

1 cup cucumber,
mushrooms, and/or other
high-volume veggies
(page 345)

2 large hard-boiled egg
whites, sliced

1 tablespoon crumbled
reduced-fat feta cheese

2 tablespoons salsa
or pico de gallo with
90mg sodium or less per
2-tablespoon serving

2 teaspoons balsamic,
red wine, or white wine
vinegar

7. Plate tofu and tomato. Sprinkle tofu and veggies with garlic powder, onion powder, and black pepper. Drizzle with any remaining balsamic vinegar.

8. Toss salad ingredients in a medium bowl, and serve alongside tofu and veggies.

MAKES 1 SERVING

Eggplant & Ricotta Tower
with side salad

Entire recipe: 335 calories, 9g fat, 712mg sodium, 35g carbs, 11.5g fiber, 16.5g sugars, 31.5g protein

TOWER

Three ½-inch-thick eggplant slices (cut widthwise from the center of a medium eggplant)

2 large tomato slices

⅛ teaspoon garlic powder

⅛ teaspoon onion powder

⅓ cup light/low-fat ricotta cheese

2 tablespoons shredded part-skim mozzarella cheese

⅛ teaspoon each salt and black pepper

⅓ cup chopped onion

2 cups chopped spinach leaves

1 teaspoon chopped garlic

1 tablespoon balsamic vinegar

(continued on next page)

You'll Need: grill pan, nonstick spray, plate, 2 medium bowls, skillet

Prep: 10 minutes

Cook: 30 minutes

1. Bring a grill pan sprayed with nonstick spray to medium-high heat. Grill eggplant until softened and slightly charred, about 8 minutes per side.

2. Transfer eggplant to a plate. Grill tomato slices until softened and slightly charred, about 2 minutes per side.

3. Transfer tomato to the plate. Season eggplant and tomato with garlic powder and onion powder. Cover to keep warm.

4. In a medium bowl, combine ricotta cheese, mozzarella cheese, salt, and pepper. Mix well.

5. Bring a skillet sprayed with nonstick spray to medium-high heat. Cook and stir onion until softened, about 4 minutes. Add spinach and chopped garlic. Cook until spinach has wilted, about 1 minute. Remove from heat, and blot away excess moisture.

SIDE SALAD

1 cup lettuce

¼ cup frozen shelled ready-to-eat edamame (unsalted), thawed

3 chopped hard-boiled egg whites

2 teaspoons vinegar (balsamic, red wine, white wlne, rice, or cider)

6. Stir spinach mixture into ricotta mixture.

7. Top one eggplant slice with half of the spinach-ricotta mixture. Repeat layering with remaining eggplant slice and spinach-ricotta mixture. Top with tomato slices, and drizzle with balsamic vinegar.

8. Toss salad ingredients in a medium bowl, and serve alongside your veggie stack.

MAKES 1 SERVING

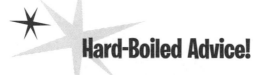

Hard-Boiled Advice!

For a step-by-step guide to hard-boiling egg whites—plus a super list of swaps—flip to page 323!

Tacos, Tostadas, and More

Soft tacos, crunchy tacos, Mexican tostadas, not-so-Mexican tostadas . . . This chapter is bursting with flavorful meals. Feel like having eggs for dinner? There's a tostada for that!

Shrimp Soft Tacos 📷

Entire recipe: 350 calories, 9.5g fat, 737mg sodium, 34.5g carbs, 5.5g fiber, 4g sugars, 30g protein

4½ ounces (about 8) raw large shrimp, peeled, tails removed, deveined

1 teaspoon taco seasoning mix

1 teaspoon lime juice

1 teaspoon olive oil or grapeseed oil

Two 6-inch corn tortillas

1½ tablespoons light sour cream

¼ cup shredded lettuce

¼ cup canned black beans or pinto beans, drained and rinsed

2 tablespoons chopped cilantro

You'll Need: skillet, nonstick spray, microwave-safe plate

Prep: 5 minutes

Cook: 5 minutes

1. Bring a skillet sprayed with nonstick spray to medium heat. Add shrimp, taco seasoning, lime juice, and oil. Cook and stir for about 4 minutes, until shrimp are cooked through.

2. On a microwave-safe plate, microwave tortillas for 15 seconds, or until warm.

3. Spread sour cream down the center of each tortilla. Top with lettuce, beans, shrimp mixture, and cilantro. Fold 'em up.

MAKES 1 SERVING

Chicken Crunchy Tacos *with side salad*

Entire recipe: 342 calories, 11g fat, 512mg sodium, 31.5g carbs, 4.5g fiber, 7.5g sugars, 30g protein

TACOS

One 3.5-ounce raw boneless skinless chicken breast cutlet, pounded to ½-inch thickness

½ teaspoon taco seasoning mix

2 corn taco shells (flat-bottomed, if available)

¼ cup shredded lettuce

2 tablespoons shredded reduced-fat Mexican-blend cheese

2 tablespoons salsa or pico de gallo with 90mg sodium or less per 2-tablespoon serving

SIDE SALAD

1 cup lettuce

1 cup cucumber, mushrooms, and/or other high-volume veggies (page 345)

2 tablespoons salsa or pico de gallo with 90mg sodium or less per 2-tablespoon serving

2 teaspoons vinegar (balsamic, red wine, white wine, rice, or cider)

You'll Need: skillet, nonstick spray, medium bowl, small bowl

Prep: 10 minutes

Cook: 10 minutes

1. Bring a skillet sprayed with nonstick spray to medium heat. Cook chicken for about 4 minutes per side, until cooked through.

2. Transfer chicken to a medium bowl. Shred using two forks—one to hold the chicken in place, and the other to scrape across the meat and shred it.

3. In a small bowl, mix taco seasoning with ½ teaspoon water. Add to the chicken, and toss to coat.

4. Divide chicken between taco shells, and top with lettuce, cheese, and salsa/pico de gallo.

5. Assemble side salad in a medium bowl, and serve with tacos.

MAKES 1 SERVING

Veggie-Friendly Soft Tacos

Entire recipe: 342 calories, 7.5g fat, 698mg sodium, 42g carbs, 11g fiber, 5.5g sugars, 34.5g protein

2 tablespoons fat-free plain Greek yogurt

2 tablespoons salsa or pico de gallo with 90mg sodium or less per 2-tablespoon serving

1¼ cups frozen ground-beef-style soy crumbles

¼ teaspoon ground cumin

¼ teaspoon chili powder

¼ teaspoon garlic powder

⅛ teaspoon onion powder

Two 6-inch corn tortillas

2 tablespoons shredded reduced-fat Mexican-blend cheese

¼ cup shredded lettuce

2 tablespoons chopped onion

You'll Need: small bowl, skillet, nonstick spray, microwave-safe plate

Prep: 10 minutes

Cook: 5 minutes

1. In a small bowl, mix yogurt with salsa/pico de gallo until uniform.

2. Bring a skillet sprayed with nonstick spray to medium-high heat. Add soy crumbles, and sprinkle with seasonings. Cook and stir until hot, about 4 minutes.

3. On a microwave-safe plate, microwave tortillas for 15 seconds, or until warm.

4. Spread yogurt-salsa mixture down the center of the tortillas. Top with cooked soy crumbles, cheese, lettuce, and onion. Fold 'em up.

MAKES 1 SERVING

Cheeseburger Tostadas

Entire recipe: 350 calories, 10g fat, 654mg sodium, 30g carbs, 3g fiber, 7g sugars, 32g protein

Two 6-inch corn tortillas

4 ounces raw extra-lean ground beef (4% fat or less)

½ cup finely chopped brown mushrooms

Dash garlic powder

Dash onion powder

Dash black pepper

1 wedge The Laughing Cow Light Creamy Swiss cheese

1½ tablespoons shredded reduced-fat cheddar cheese

2 tablespoons chopped tomato

2 tablespoons finely chopped onion

1 tablespoon chopped dill pickle

2 teaspoons ketchup

1 teaspoon yellow mustard

You'll Need: baking sheet, nonstick spray, skillet

Prep: 10 minutes

Cook: 10 minutes

1. Preheat oven to 375 degrees. Spray a baking sheet with nonstick spray.

2. Lay tortillas on the sheet, and spray with nonstick spray. Bake for 5 minutes.

3. Flip tortillas, and bake until crispy, 3 to 4 minutes.

4. Meanwhile, bring a skillet sprayed with nonstick spray to medium-high heat. Add beef, mushrooms, and seasonings. Cook, stir, and crumble until beef is fully cooked and mushrooms have softened, 3 to 4 minutes. Add cheese wedge, breaking it into pieces. Cook and stir until cheese has melted and is evenly distributed, about 1 minute.

5. Divide beef mixture between baked tortillas, and sprinkle with shredded cheese. Top with tomato, onion, pickle, ketchup, and mustard.

MAKES 1 SERVING

Have Leftover Corn Tortillas? Make DIY Tortilla Chips!

Here's how to make a 100-calorie batch . . . an HG-Diet-approved snack!

Preheat oven to 400 degrees. Spray a baking sheet lightly with nonstick spray.

Cut 2 corn tortillas in half. Cut each half into 3 triangles, for a total of 12 triangles.

Place tortilla triangles close together on the sheet. Spray with nonstick spray, and sprinkle with a dash of salt.

Bake for 5 minutes. Carefully flip triangles and bake until crispy, 2 to 4 minutes.

For a sweet spin, don't miss the Churro Chips 'n Dip on page 282!

Breakfast for Dinner Tostadas

Entire recipe: 336 calories, 8.5g fat, 721mg sodium, 32g carbs, 6g fiber, 4.5g sugars, 31g protein

Two 6-inch corn tortillas

2 tablespoons chopped onion

¾ cup egg whites or fat-free liquid egg substitute

1¾ ounces (about 4 slices) chopped reduced-sodium ham

¼ cup chopped tomato

1½ ounces (about 3 tablespoons) chopped avocado

1 tablespoon chopped cilantro

⅛ teaspoon garlic powder

⅛ teaspoon onion powder

⅛ teaspoon chili powder

You'll Need: baking sheet, nonstick spray, large microwave-safe mug, small bowl

Prep: 5 minutes

Cook: 10 minutes

1. Preheat oven to 375 degrees. Spray a baking sheet with nonstick spray.

2. Lay tortillas on the sheet, and spray with nonstick spray. Bake for 5 minutes.

3. Flip tortillas, and bake until crispy, 3 to 4 minutes.

4. Meanwhile, spray a large microwave-safe mug with nonstick spray. Microwave onion for 30 seconds, or until softened. Add egg whites/substitute, and microwave for 1 minute. Stir in ham, and microwave for 1 minute, or until set.

5. Divide egg scramble between baked tortillas.

6. In a small bowl, mix remaining ingredients. Spoon over egg scramble.

MAKES 1 SERVING

Caesar Salad Tostadas

Entire recipe: 350 calories, 10.5g fat, 620mg sodium, 28.5g carbs, 4g fiber, 4.5g sugars, 35g protein

Two 6-inch corn tortillas

1 stick light string cheese

3 ounces cooked and finely chopped skinless chicken breast

3 tablespoons finely chopped red onion

1 cup finely chopped romaine lettuce

1 tablespoon light Caesar dressing

3 tablespoons chopped tomato

2 teaspoons grated Parmesan cheese

You'll Need: baking sheet, nonstick spray, blender or food processor (optional), medium bowl

Prep: 10 minutes

Cook: 10 minutes

1. Preheat oven to 375 degrees. Spray a baking sheet with nonstick spray.

2. Lay tortillas on the sheet, and spray with nonstick spray. Bake for 5 minutes.

3. Meanwhile, break string cheese into thirds and place in blender or food processor—blend at high speed until shredded. (Or pull into shreds and roughly chop.)

4. Flip tortillas. Top with shredded string cheese, chicken, and red onion. Bake until tortillas are crispy and cheese has melted, 3 to 4 minutes.

5. Meanwhile, in a medium bowl, toss lettuce with dressing.

6. Divide lettuce mixture between baked tortillas, top with tomato, and sprinkle with Parm.

MAKES 1 SERVING

Greek Salad Tostada 📷

Entire recipe: 330 calories, 7.5g fat, 716mg sodium, 37g carbs, 8.5g fiber, 8g sugars, 35g protein

1 medium-large high-fiber flour tortilla with 110 calories or less

2 tablespoons fat-free plain Greek yogurt

Drop lemon juice

Dash black pepper

Dash dried oregano

3 ounces cooked and chopped skinless chicken breast

¾ cup chopped cucumber

¼ cup chopped red onion

½ cup shredded lettuce

½ cup halved cherry tomatoes

2 tablespoons crumbled reduced-fat feta cheese

1 tablespoon canned sliced black olives, drained

You'll Need: baking sheet, nonstick spray, medium bowl

Prep: 10 minutes

Cook: 10 minutes

1. Preheat oven to 375 degrees. Spray a baking sheet with nonstick spray.

2. Lay tortilla on the sheet, and bake until slightly crispy, about 5 minutes.

3. Meanwhile, in a medium bowl, combine yogurt, lemon juice, pepper, and oregano. Mix well. Add chicken, cucumber, and onion. Stir to coat.

4. Flip tortilla. Bake until crispy, about 3 minutes.

5. Top baked tortilla with lettuce, tomatoes, chicken mixture, feta cheese, and olives.

MAKES 1 SERVING

Need Chicken Cooking Tips?

Check out page 319, or purchase precooked chicken!

Breakfast-Style Burrito Crepes

Entire recipe: 349 calories, 6.5g fat, 684mg sodium, 34g carbs, 5.5g fiber, 11g sugars, 39.5g protein

½ cup egg whites

1½ tablespoons plain protein powder with about 100 calories per serving

½ cup chopped green bell pepper

⅓ cup frozen sweet corn kernels

¼ cup chopped onion

¼ cup canned black beans, drained and rinsed

¼ cup shredded reduced-fat Mexican-blend cheese

⅓ cup fat-free plain Greek yogurt

1½ tablespoons salsa or pico de gallo with 90mg sodium or less per 2-tablespoon serving

You'll Need: 2 small bowls, whisk, 10-inch skillet, nonstick spray, offset spatula or flexible rubber spatula, plate

Prep: 10 minutes

Cook: 15 minutes

1. To make the batter, in a small bowl, combine egg whites with protein powder. Whisk until uniform.

2. To make the crepes, bring a 10-inch skillet sprayed with nonstick spray to medium heat. Pour half of the batter into the pan, quickly tilting the skillet in all directions to evenly coat the bottom. Cook until lightly browned on the bottom, about 2 minutes. Carefully flip with an offset spatula or flexible rubber spatula. Cook until lightly browned on the other side, about 1 minute.

3. Transfer the crepe to a plate, and repeat with remaining egg mixture to make another crepe. Cover to keep warm.

4. Remove skillet from heat; clean, if needed. Re-spray, and return to medium heat. Add pepper, corn, and onion. Cook and stir until slightly softened and lightly browned, about 4 minutes. Add beans, and cook and stir until hot, about 1 minute. Evenly divide between the centers of the crepes.

5. Sprinkle with cheese, and wrap crepes around the filling.

6. In a second small bowl, mix yogurt with salsa/pico de gallo until uniform. Spoon over stuffed crepes.

MAKES 1 SERVING

HG FYI

Flip to page 80 for crepe tips 'n tricks!

Turkey Avocado Burrito

Entire recipe: 340 calories, 10g fat, 749mg sodium, 40.5g carbs, 11.5g fiber, 4.5g sugars, 30g protein

3 ounces raw lean ground turkey (7% fat or less)

⅛ teaspoon ground cumin

⅛ teaspoon garlic powder

⅛ teaspoon chili powder

Dash each salt and black pepper

2 tablespoons fat-free plain Greek yogurt

½ ounce (about 1 tablespoon) mashed avocado

1 tablespoon canned green chiles, lightly drained

1 medium-large high-fiber flour tortilla with 110 calories or less

½ cup shredded lettuce

¼ cup chopped tomato

¼ cup canned black beans, drained and rinsed

You'll Need: skillet, nonstick spray, small bowl, microwave-safe plate

Prep: 10 minutes

Cook: 5 minutes

1. Bring a skillet sprayed with nonstick spray to medium-high heat. Add turkey, and sprinkle with seasonings. Cook and crumble for about 3 minutes, until fully cooked.

2. In a small bowl, mix Greek yogurt with avocado until uniform. Stir in green chiles.

3. Microwave tortilla on a microwave-safe plate for 10 seconds, or until warm.

4. Spread yogurt mixture down the center of the tortilla. Top with lettuce, tomato, beans, and cooked turkey.

5. Wrap up tortilla by first folding one side in (to keep filling from escaping), and then rolling it up from the bottom.

MAKES 1 SERVING

Shrimp Fajitas

Entire recipe: 349 calories, 7.5g fat, 715mg sodium, 40.5g carbs, 6.5g fiber, 8.5g sugars, 32.5g protein

1 portabella mushroom, sliced

⅓ cup sliced bell pepper

⅓ cup sliced onion

1 teaspoon olive oil or grapeseed oil

4 ounces (about 7) raw large shrimp, peeled, tails removed, deveined

2 teaspoons fajita seasoning mix

1 teaspoon lime juice

Two 6-inch corn tortillas

1 cup shredded lettuce

¼ cup diced tomato

2 tablespoons fat-free plain Greek yogurt

You'll Need: large skillet, nonstick spray, microwave-safe plate

Prep: 10 minutes

Cook: 10 minutes

1. Bring a large skillet sprayed with nonstick spray to medium-high heat. Add sliced mushroom, pepper, and onion, and drizzle with oil. Cook and stir until mostly softened, about 5 minutes.

2. Add shrimp, seasoning mix, lime juice, and 2 tablespoons water. Cook and stir until veggies have softened and shrimp are cooked through, about 2 minutes.

3. Microwave tortillas on a microwave-safe plate for 10 seconds, or until warm. Top tortillas with lettuce, shrimp mixture, tomato, and yogurt. Fold 'em up.

MAKES 1 SERVING

Soups, Stews & Bowls

Who doesn't love a giant bowl of DELICIOUS? These meals are super filling and packed with flavor. (Pssst . . . The Cioppino à la HG is a favorite here at Hungryland!)

Cioppino à la HG

½ of recipe (about 2¼ cups): 335 calories, 8.5g fat, 714mg sodium, 28g carbs, 3.5g fiber, 12g sugars, 36.5g protein

¾ cup chopped onion

½ cup chopped bell pepper

2 teaspoons olive oil or grapeseed oil

1 teaspoon chopped garlic

One 14.5-ounce can creamy reduced-sodium tomato soup with 4g fat or less per cup

1½ cups low-sodium vegetable broth

¼ teaspoon paprika

6 ounces (about 10) raw large shrimp, peeled, tails removed, and deveined, chopped

6 ounces raw tilapia, cod, or sea bass, cut into bite-sized pieces

2 tablespoons finely chopped cilantro

Optional seasonings: salt-free seasoning mix, red pepper flakes

You'll Need: medium-large pot, nonstick spray

Prep: 15 minutes

Cook: 15 minutes

1. Bring a medium-large pot sprayed with nonstick spray to medium-high heat. Add onion and pepper, and drizzle with oil. Cook and stir until slightly softened and lightly browned, about 4 minutes. Add garlic, and cook and stir until fragrant, about 1 minute.

2. Carefully add soup, broth, and paprika. Bring to a boil.

3. Reduce to a simmer. Add shrimp and fish. Stirring occasionally, cook for about 4 minutes, until fish and shrimp are just cooked through. Top with cilantro.

MAKES 2 SERVINGS

Mexican Taco Soup

Entire recipe: 350 calories, 11.5g fat, 669mg sodium, 29g carbs, 4g fiber, 7g sugars, 33.5g protein

½ cup chopped celery

2 tablespoons chopped onion

4 ounces raw extra-lean ground beef (4% fat or less)

1 teaspoon chopped garlic

1 teaspoon taco seasoning mix

2 cups low-sodium beef, chicken, or vegetable broth

½ cup chopped tomato

¼ cup frozen sweet corn kernels

1 teaspoon salt-free seasoning mix

1 corn taco shell

2 tablespoons shredded reduced-fat Mexican-blend cheese

Optional seasoning: cayenne pepper

Optional topping: chopped cilantro

You'll Need: medium pot with a lid, nonstick spray, large bowl

Prep: 10 minutes

Cook: 20 minutes

1. Bring a medium pot sprayed with nonstick spray to medium heat. Add celery and onion. Cook and stir until browned, about 4 minutes. Add beef, garlic, and ½ teaspoon taco seasoning, and cook and crumble until veggies have softened and beef is fully cooked, about 3 minutes.

2. Carefully add broth, tomato, corn, salt-free seasoning, and remaining ½ teaspoon taco seasoning. Bring to a boil, and then reduce to a simmer.

3. Cover and cook for 10 minutes, or until veggies are soft. Transfer to a large bowl.

4. Lightly crush taco shell, and distribute over the soup. Sprinkle with cheese.

MAKES 1 SERVING

Chicken Noodle Bowl 📷

½ of recipe (about 4¼ cups): 348 calories, 8.5g fat, 678mg sodium, 31.5g carbs, 12g fiber, 9.5g sugars, 39.5g protein

3 bags House Foods Tofu Shirataki Fettuccine Shaped Noodle Substitute

1 cup chopped celery

1 cup chopped carrots

¾ cup chopped onion

2 teaspoons olive oil or grapeseed oil

1 teaspoon salt-free seasoning mix, or more to taste

3½ cups low-sodium chicken broth

2 cups bagged cole slaw mix

¼ teaspoon ground thyme

1 dried bay leaf

10 ounces raw boneless skinless chicken breast

¼ teaspoon each salt and black pepper

½ cup frozen peas

You'll Need: strainer, large pot, nonstick spray, large bowl

Prep: 15 minutes

Cook: 30 minutes

1. Use a strainer to rinse and drain noodles. Thoroughly pat dry. Roughly cut noodles.

2. Bring a large pot sprayed with nonstick spray to medium-high heat. Add celery, carrots, and onion. Drizzle with oil, and sprinkle with salt-free seasoning. Cook and stir until browned and softened, about 8 minutes.

3. Carefully add broth to the pot. Add noodles, cole slaw mix, thyme, and bay leaf.

4. Season chicken with ⅛ teaspoon each salt and pepper. Add to the pot, submerging it completely. Bring to a boil.

5. Reduce to a simmer. Cook for about 12 minutes, until chicken is cooked through.

6. Remove and discard bay leaf. Transfer chicken to a large bowl. Shred with two forks—one to hold the chicken in place and the other to scrape across and shred it.

7. Add shredded chicken, peas, and remaining ⅛ teaspoon each salt and pepper to the pot. Cook and stir until and peas are hot, about 2 minutes.

MAKES 2 SERVINGS

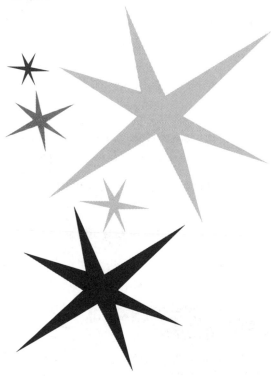

Chicken Chili 📷

Entire recipe: 344 calories, 6.5g fat, 665mg sodium, 33g carbs, 8.5g fiber, 11.5g sugars, 38.5g protein

¼ cup chopped onion

1 tablespoon chopped jalapeño pepper

4 ounces raw boneless skinless chicken breast, cut into ½-inch cubes

¾ teaspoon chili powder

¼ teaspoon ground cumin

¼ cup chopped tomato

½ teaspoon crushed garlic

⅔ cup canned crushed tomatoes

¼ cup canned black beans or pinto beans, drained and rinsed

1 tablespoon tomato paste

2 tablespoons shredded reduced-fat cheddar cheese

1 tablespoon fat-free plain Greek yogurt

You'll Need: medium pot, nonstick spray

Prep: 15 minutes

Cook: 15 minutes

1. Bring a medium pot sprayed with nonstick spray to medium-high heat. Add onion and jalapeño pepper. Cook and stir until browned, about 2 minutes.

2. Add chicken to the pot, and season with ¼ teaspoon chili powder and ⅛ teaspoon cumin. Cook and stir for about 4 minutes, until cooked through.

3. Add chopped tomato and garlic. Cook and stir until garlic is fragrant, about 1 minute.

4. Carefully add crushed tomatoes, beans, and tomato paste. Add remaining ½ teaspoon chili powder and remaining ⅛ teaspoon cumin, and mix thoroughly.

5. Cook and stir until hot and well mixed, about 3 minutes.

6. Serve topped with cheese and yogurt.

MAKES 1 SERVING

HG Tip!

When handling jalapeños, don't touch your eyes—that pepper juice can STING. And wash your hands well immediately afterward.

Chopped Greek Salad Bowl

Entire recipe: 330 calories, 7.5g fat, 694mg sodium, 36g carbs, 9g fiber, 14g sugars, 32.5g protein

2 cups chopped iceberg or romaine lettuce

⅓ cup fat-free plain Greek yogurt

2 teaspoons lemon juice

⅛ teaspoon dried oregano

⅛ teaspoon garlic powder

⅛ teaspoon onion powder

1 cup chopped cucumber

1 cup chopped tomato

⅓ cup canned garbanzo beans/chickpeas, drained and rinsed

¼ cup chopped red onion

¼ cup crumbled reduced-fat feta cheese

3 hard-boiled egg whites, chopped

You'll Need: 2 medium-large bowls

Prep: 15 minutes

1. Place lettuce in a medium-large bowl.

2. In another medium-large bowl, combine yogurt, lemon juice, and seasonings. Mix well. Add remaining ingredients, and toss to coat. Serve over lettuce.

MAKES 1 SERVING

For the latest food news, recipes, tips 'n tricks, and more, **sign up for free daily emails at hungry-girl.com!**

Shrimp Quinoa Veggie Bowl

Entire recipe: 345 calories, 8g fat, 607g sodium, 33.5g carbs, 4g fiber, 5g sugars, 33.5g protein

1 cup roughly chopped spinach leaves

3 tablespoons uncooked quinoa, rinsed thoroughly

1 teaspoon chopped garlic

¾ cup chopped brown mushrooms

¼ cup chopped onion

5 ounces (about 9) raw large shrimp, peeled, tails removed, deveined

2 teaspoons balsamic vinegar

1 teaspoon olive oil or grapeseed oil

Dash each salt and black pepper

You'll Need: medium-large bowl, small nonstick pot, skillet, nonstick spray

Prep: 10 minutes

Cook: 20 minutes

1. Place spinach in a medium-large bowl.

2. In a small nonstick pot, combine quinoa, garlic, and ⅓ cup water. Bring to a boil.

3. Reduce heat to low. Cover and simmer for 10 minutes, or until water has been absorbed and quinoa is fully cooked. Transfer to the bowl, and cover to keep warm.

4. Bring a skillet sprayed with nonstick spray to medium-high heat. Add mushrooms and onion. Cook and stir until mostly softened, about 2 minutes.

5. Add shrimp to the skillet. Cook and stir for about 3 minutes, until cooked through.

6. Transfer contents of the skillet to the bowl. Add remaining ingredients, and mix well.

MAKES 1 SERVING

Super-Savory Quinoa Bowl

Entire recipe: 350 calories, 9g fat, 658mg sodium, 40.5g carbs, 10.5g fiber, 4.5g sugars, 33g protein

1½ cups roughly chopped spinach leaves

3 tablespoons uncooked quinoa, rinsed thoroughly

½ teaspoon chopped garlic

1 cup sliced mushrooms

1 cup frozen ground-beef-style soy crumbles

1½ teaspoons light whipped butter or light buttery spread

1 wedge The Laughing Cow Light Creamy Swiss cheese

2 tablespoons fat-free plain Greek yogurt

Dash black pepper

You'll Need: medium-large bowl, small nonstick pot, skillet, nonstick spray

Prep: 5 minutes

Cook: 20 minutes

1. Place spinach in a medium-large bowl.

2. In a small nonstick pot, combine quinoa, garlic, and ⅓ cup water. Bring to a boil.

3. Reduce heat to low. Cover and simmer for 10 minutes, or until water has absorbed and quinoa is fully cooked. Transfer to the bowl, and cover to keep warm.

4. Meanwhile, bring a skillet sprayed with nonstick spray to medium-high heat. Cook and stir mushrooms until browned and mostly softened, about 4 minutes. Add soy crumbles, and cook and stir until hot, about 2 minutes.

5. Reduce skillet heat to low. Stir in butter and cheese wedge, breaking the wedge into pieces. Cook and stir until cheese has melted, mixed with butter, and coated soy-crumble mixture, about 1 minute.

6. Transfer contents of the skillet to the bowl. Add yogurt and pepper, and mix well.

MAKES 1 SERVING

Hawaiian Beef Bowl

Entire recipe: 345 calories, 8g fat, 742mg sodium, 31g carbs, 4.5g fiber, 20.5g sugars, 36g protein

1 cup sugar snap peas

1 cup sliced bell pepper

⅓ cup sliced onion

5 ounces thinly sliced raw lean beefsteak

Dash each salt and black pepper

⅓ cup canned crushed pineapple packed in juice

2 tablespoons teriyaki sauce or marinade with 25 calories or less per tablespoon

You'll Need: large skillet, nonstick spray

Prep: 10 minutes

Cook: 10 minutes

1. Bring a large skillet sprayed with nonstick spray to medium-high heat. Add snap peas, bell pepper, and onion. Cook and stir until partially softened, about 4 minutes.

2. Add beef to the skillet, and season with salt and black pepper. Add pineapple and teriyaki sauce/marinade. Cook and stir until veggies have softened and beef is cooked through, about 3 minutes.

MAKES 1 SERVING

HG Tip!

Freeze your beef fillet slightly before cutting into it; this will make it easier to slice!

Fajita Tofu Bowl 📷

Entire recipe: 338 calories, 9g fat, 742mg sodium, 35g carbs, 8g fiber, 8g sugars, 30g protein

5 ounces block-style extra-firm tofu, cut into 1-inch cubes

⅛ teaspoon onion powder

⅛ teaspoon chili powder

Dash each salt and black pepper

1½ cups sliced brown mushrooms

¼ cup sliced onion

¼ cup sliced bell pepper

½ cup canned black beans, drained and rinsed

1¼ teaspoons fajita seasoning mix

3 tablespoons fat-free plain Greek yogurt

1 tablespoon salsa or pico de gallo with 90mg sodium or less per 2-tablespoon serving

1 tablespoon chopped cilantro

You'll Need: large skillet, nonstick spray, medium-large bowl

Prep: 10 minutes

Cook: 15 minutes

1. Bring a large skillet sprayed with nonstick spray to high heat. Season tofu with onion powder, chili powder, salt, and black pepper. Cook until golden brown, about 5 minutes, gently flipping to evenly cook.

2. Transfer tofu to a medium-large bowl, and cover to keep warm.

3. Remove skillet from heat; clean, if needed. Re-spray, and bring to medium-high heat. Add mushrooms, onion, and bell pepper. Cook and stir until softened and browned, about 5 minutes.

4. Add beans to the skillet. Sprinkle with fajita seasoning, and add 1 tablespoon water. Cook and stir until liquid has thickened and coated veggies, about 1 minute. Transfer to the bowl, and gently stir to mix.

5. Top with yogurt, salsa/pico de gallo, and cilantro.

MAKES 1 SERVING

BBQ Chicken Bowl

Entire recipe: 342 calories, 9g fat, 501mg sodium, 34g carbs, 8.5g fiber, 17.5g sugars, 33.5g protein

2 cups shredded lettuce

1⅓ cups chopped bell pepper

⅓ cup chopped onion

4½ ounces raw boneless skinless chicken breast, cut into bite-sized pieces

Dash each salt and black pepper

2 tablespoons frozen sweet corn kernels

1½ tablespoons BBQ sauce with 45 calories or less per 2-tablespoon serving

1½ teaspoons light sour cream

1 ounce (about 2 tablespoons) chopped avocado

You'll Need: medium-large bowl, skillet, nonstick spray

Prep: 15 minutes

Cook: 10 minutes

1. Place lettuce in a medium-large bowl.

2. Bring a skillet sprayed with nonstick spray to medium-high heat. Add bell pepper and onion. Cook and stir until partially softened, about 3 minutes.

3. Add chicken to the skillet, and season with salt and black pepper. Add corn, and cook and stir until veggies have slightly browned and chicken is fully cooked, about 4 minutes.

4. Remove skillet from heat. Add BBQ sauce and sour cream, and stir until well mixed and evenly distributed. Let cool slightly.

5. Transfer contents of the skillet to the bowl. Top with avocado.

MAKES 1 SERVING

Salads

Break out your biggest bowls, because these ginormous salads are here to satisfy! These meals also travel really well.

Tremendous Taco Salad

Entire recipe: 350 calories, 9.5g fat, 414mg sodium, 35.5g carbs, 8g fiber, 9.5g sugars, 31.5g protein

3 cups shredded lettuce

1 cup bagged cole slaw mix

2 teaspoons lime juice

4 ounces raw extra-lean ground beef (4% fat or less)

½ cup finely chopped brown mushrooms

¼ cup chopped onion

1 teaspoon taco seasoning mix

2 tablespoons canned black beans, drained and rinsed

2 tablespoons frozen sweet corn kernels

¼ cup chopped tomato

1 corn taco shell, lightly crushed

1 tablespoon light sour cream

You'll Need: large bowl, skillet, nonstick spray

Prep: 10 minutes

Cook: 10 minutes

1. Place lettuce and cole slaw mix in a large bowl. Add lime juice, and toss to coat.

2. Bring a skillet sprayed with nonstick spray to medium-high heat. Add beef, mushrooms, and onion. Cook, stir, and crumble until beef is fully cooked and veggies have softened, about 4 minutes.

3. Sprinkle with taco seasoning, and continue to cook until excess moisture has evaporated, about 1 minute.

4. Add black beans and corn, and cook and stir until hot, about 2 minutes.

5. Transfer contents of the skillet to the bowl. Top with tomato, crushed taco shell, and sour cream.

MAKES 1 SERVING

Buffalo Chicken Salad

Entire recipe: 330 calories, 7.5g fat, 750mg sodium, 32g carbs, 12.5g fiber, 15g sugars, 39g protein

SALAD

4 cups chopped romaine or iceberg lettuce

1 cup chopped celery

1 cup chopped carrots

¾ cup chopped tomato

4 ounces cooked and chopped skinless chicken breast

1 teaspoon Frank's RedHot Original Cayenne Pepper Sauce

DRESSING

2½ tablespoons fat-free plain Greek yogurt

1 ounce (about 2 tablespoons) mashed avocado

¾ teaspoon ranch dressing/dip seasoning mix

You'll Need: large bowl, medium bowl, small bowl

Prep: 10 minutes

1. In a large bowl, combine all salad ingredients *except* chicken and hot sauce.

2. Place chicken in a medium bowl. Add hot sauce, and stir to coat. Top salad with chicken mixture.

3. Combine dressing ingredients in a small bowl. And 1½ tablespoons water, and stir until uniform. Top salad with dressing, or serve dressing on the side.

MAKES 1 SERVING

Time-Saving Salad Shortcut

Instead of chopping up romaine or iceberg lettuce, go for bagged, pre-chopped salad greens. Just avoid the heavy add-ins, like nuts, dried fruit, and croutons. Extra veggies are A-OK, though!

BBQ Shrimp Salad

Entire recipe: 344 calories, 9g fat, 736mg sodium, 34g carbs, 11.5g fiber, 10.5g sugars, 35g protein

SALAD

4 cups chopped romaine or iceberg lettuce

¼ cup chopped tomato

¼ cup chopped jicama

4 ounces ready-to-eat shrimp

1½ ounces (about 3 tablespoons) chopped avocado

3 tablespoons canned black beans, drained and rinsed

3 tablespoons frozen sweet corn kernels, thawed

1 tablespoon chopped cilantro

DRESSING

1 tablespoon BBQ sauce with 45 calories or less per 2-tablespoon serving

1 tablespoon fat-free plain Greek yogurt

¾ teaspoon ranch dressing/dip seasoning mix

You'll Need: large bowl, small bowl

Prep: 10 minutes

1. Place all salad ingredients in a large bowl.

2. Combine dressing ingredients in a small bowl. Add 2 teaspoons water, and stir until uniform. Drizzle over salad, or serve on the side.

MAKES 1 SERVING

Thai Tuna Salad

Entire recipe: 340 calories, 7.5g fat, 519mg sodium, 41g carbs, 13g fiber, 24g sugars, 35g protein

SALAD

4 cups chopped romaine or iceberg lettuce

2 cups bean sprouts

1½ cups roughly chopped snap peas

1 cup sliced mushrooms

2 tablespoons chopped cilantro

2 tablespoons chopped scallions

One 2.6-ounce pouch low-sodium tuna packed in water, flaked

DRESSING

1 tablespoon plain rice vinegar

2 teaspoons creamy peanut butter

1 teaspoon reduced-sodium/lite soy sauce

1 teaspoon Sriracha sauce

1 teaspoon granulated white sugar

You'll Need: large bowl, medium bowl, whisk

Prep: 10 minutes

1. Place all salad ingredients in a large bowl.

2. In a medium bowl, combine all dressing ingredients. Add 1 tablespoon water, and whisk until dressing is uniform and sugar has dissolved. Drizzle over salad, or serve on the side.

MAKES 1 SERVING

Fruit 'n Tuna Salad

Entire recipe: 342 calories, 9g fat, 647mg sodium, 32.5g carbs, 5.5g fiber, 22g sugars, 34g protein

4 cups chopped romaine or iceberg lettuce

1½ tablespoons light mayonnaise

1 tablespoon fat-free plain Greek yogurt

Dash each salt and black pepper

4 ounces low-sodium tuna packed in water (drained)

¼ cup chopped apple

¼ cup halved red seedless grapes

¼ cup chopped cucumber

1 tablespoon sweetened dried cranberries

2 tablespoons low-fat balsamic vinaigrette

You'll Need: large bowl, medium bowl

Prep: 15 minutes

1. Place lettuce in a large bowl.

2. In a medium bowl, combine mayo, yogurt, salt, and pepper. Mix well. Add all remaining ingredients *except* vinaigrette. Stir to coat.

3. Add tuna mixture to the large bowl. Drizzle with vinaigrette, or serve vinaigrette on the side.

MAKES 1 SERVING

Cranberry Kale Chicken Salad 📷

Entire recipe: 344 calories, 8.5g fat, 507mg sodium, 33.5g carbs, 5.5g fiber, 19.5g sugars, 36g protein

1 cup chopped kale leaves

½ cup sliced apple

½ cup thinly sliced cucumber

½ cup carrot sliced into coins

1 tablespoon lemon juice

4 ounces cooked and shredded (or roughly chopped) skinless chicken breast

2 tablespoons fat-free plain Greek yogurt

1½ tablespoons sweetened dried cranberries

¼ ounce (about 1 tablespoon) sliced almonds

2 teaspoons light mayonnaise

⅛ teaspoon garlic powder

Dash each salt and black pepper

You'll Need: large bowl, medium bowl

Prep: 10 minutes

1. In a large bowl, combine kale, apple, cucumber, carrots, and lemon juice. Mix well.

2. In a medium bowl, combine remaining ingredients, and mix well.

3. Add chicken mixture to the large bowl.

MAKES 1 SERVING

HG Tip!

It may sound funny, but massage your kale leaves! This tenderizes them, improving the texture.

📷 Photo Alert!

The camera icon next to the recipe name means flip to the insert to see a photo of this recipe. Find full-color photos of ALL the recipes at hungry-girl.com/books.

Cheeseburger Salad

Entire recipe: 341 calories, 8g fat, 720mg sodium, 41g carbs, 14.5g fiber, 17g sugars, 35.5g protein

SALAD

4 cups shredded lettuce

1 cup chopped tomato

1 cup chopped brown mushrooms

½ cup chopped onion

1 cup frozen ground-beef-style soy crumbles

3 tablespoons Sargento Reduced Fat Sharp Cheddar shredded cheese

DRESSING

2 tablespoons fat-free plain Greek yogurt

1 tablespoon ketchup

You'll Need: large bowl, skillet, nonstick spray, small bowl

Prep: 10 minutes

Cook: 10 minutes

1. Place lettuce and tomato in a large bowl.

2. Bring a skillet sprayed with nonstick spray to medium-high heat. Add mushrooms and onion. Cook and stir until mostly softened, about 3 minutes.

3. Reduce heat to medium. Add soy crumbles, and cook and stir until hot, about 2 minutes. Remove from heat.

4. Transfer soy-crumble mixture to the large bowl, and sprinkle with cheese.

5. To make the dressing, in a small bowl, mix yogurt with ketchup until uniform. Top salad with dressing, or serve dressing on the side.

MAKES 1 SERVING

Fruity Chicken Chopped Salad

Entire recipe: 348 calories, 9.5g fat, 421mg sodium, 35g carbs, 9g fiber, 22.5g sugars, 34.5g protein

SALAD

4 cups chopped romaine or iceberg lettuce

2 cups chopped spinach leaves

4 ounces cooked and chopped skinless chicken breast

½ cup chopped peach

⅓ cup chopped pear

¼ cup blueberries

DRESSING

2 tablespoons balsamic vinegar

1½ teaspoons extra-virgin olive oil or grapeseed oil

½ teaspoon chopped garlic

Dash each salt and black pepper

You'll Need: large bowl, medium bowl, whisk

Prep: 10 minutes

1. Place salad ingredients in a large bowl.

2. In a medium bowl, combine dressing ingredients. Whisk thoroughly. Drizzle over salad, or serve on the side.

MAKES 1 SERVING

Need Chicken Cooking Tips?

Check out page 319, or purchase precooked chicken!

Tropical Shrimp Salad 📷

Entire recipe: 345 calories, 7g fat, 605mg sodium, 37g carbs, 12g fiber, 17g sugars, 38g protein

SALAD

4 cups chopped romaine or iceberg lettuce

4 ounces ready-to-eat shrimp

1 ounce (about 2 tablespoons) chopped avocado

½ cup chopped mango

⅓ cup chopped jicama

¼ cup canned black beans, drained and rinsed

DRESSING

3 tablespoons fat-free plain Greek yogurt

1 teaspoon lime juice

1 teaspoon finely chopped cilantro

⅛ teaspoon garlic powder

Dash each salt and black pepper

You'll Need: large bowl, small bowl

Prep: 10 minutes

1. Place salad ingredients in a large bowl.

2. In a small bowl, combine dressing ingredients. Add 1 tablespoon water, and mix until uniform. Drizzle over salad, or serve on the side.

MAKES 1 SERVING

Greek Tuna Salad

Entire recipe: 343 calories, 9.5g fat, 606mg sodium, 31.5g carbs, 8.5g fiber, 16.5g sugars, 37.5g protein

4 cups chopped romaine or iceberg lettuce

¼ cup fat-free plain yogurt

1½ teaspoons lemon juice

⅛ teaspoon garlic powder

⅛ teaspoon black pepper

3 ounces low-sodium tuna packed in water (drained)

1 cup chopped cucumber

1 cup cherry tomatoes, quartered

½ cup chopped red bell pepper

¼ cup chopped red onion

¼ cup crumbled reduced-fat feta cheese

2 tablespoons canned sliced black olives, drained

You'll Need: large bowl, medium-large bowl

Prep: 10 minutes

1. Place lettuce in a large bowl.

2. In a medium-large bowl, combine yogurt, lemon juice, garlic powder, and black pepper. Mix well. Add tuna, cucumber, tomatoes, bell pepper, and onion. Stir to coat.

3. Spoon tuna mixture over lettuce. Top with feta cheese and olives.

MAKES 1 SERVING

CHAPTER 9

Sandwiches, Burgers & Wraps

Ready to wrap your face around some seriously satisfying sandwiches and more handheld meals? GOOD! And definitely check out the next chapter too . . . It's full of lettuce-wrapped burgers and more lettuce-contained perfection!

Open-Faced Tuna-Egg Salad Sandwich

Entire recipe: 330 calories, 8g fat, 603mg sodium, 34.5g carbs, 8g fiber, 9g sugars, 32.5g protein

One 100-calorie flat sandwich bun *or* 2 slices light bread

2 lettuce leaves

1½ tablespoons light mayonnaise

1 tablespoon fat-free plain Greek yogurt

⅛ teaspoon onion powder

⅛ teaspoon garlic powder

Dash black pepper

One 2.6-ounce pouch low-sodium tuna packed in water

¼ cup finely chopped cucumber

¼ cup finely chopped onion

¼ cup finely chopped red bell pepper

¼ cup shredded carrots

2 hard-boiled egg whites, chopped

You'll Need: medium bowl

Prep: 10 minutes

1. If you like, lightly toast bun halves/bread slices. Top each with a lettuce leaf.

2. In a medium bowl, combine mayo, yogurt, and seasonings. Mix well. Add remaining ingredients, and stir to coat.

3. Evenly divide mixture between bun halves/bread slices.

MAKES 1 SERVING

Open-Faced Avocado-Egg Salad Sandwich

Entire recipe: 330 calories, 9g fat, 625mg sodium, 33g carbs, 9g fiber, 8g sugars, 30g protein

One 100-calorie flat sandwich bun *or* 2 slices light bread

2 lettuce leaves

2 tomato slices

1 ounce (about 2 tablespoons) roughly mashed avocado

1 tablespoon fat-free plain Greek yogurt

2½ teaspoons light mayonnaise

¼ teaspoon salt-free seasoning mix

Dash paprika

6 hard-boiled egg whites, chopped

3 tablespoons finely chopped onion

2 tablespoons finely chopped carrots

You'll Need: medium bowl

Prep: 10 minutes

1. If you like, toast bun halves/bread slices. Top each with a lettuce leaf and a tomato slice.

2. In a medium bowl, combine avocado, yogurt, mayo, salt-free seasoning, and paprika. Stir until uniform. Add remaining ingredients, and stir to coat.

3. Divide mixture between bun halves/bread slices.

MAKES 1 SERVING

Hard-Boiled Advice!

For a step-by-step guide to hard-boiling egg whites, flip to page 323!

Open-Faced Chicken Salad Sandwich
with veggies and ranch dip

Entire recipe: 345 calories, 7g fat, 692mg sodium, 36g carbs, 9g fiber, 10g sugars, 38g protein

One 100-calorie flat sandwich bun *or* 2 slices light bread

2 lettuce leaves

2 tomato slices

1 tablespoon light mayonnaise

⅛ teaspoon garlic powder

⅛ teaspoon onion powder

3 tablespoons fat-free plain Greek yogurt

3½ ounces cooked and finely chopped skinless chicken breast

2 tablespoons finely chopped celery

1 tablespoon finely chopped onion

¾ teaspoon ranch dressing/dip seasoning mix

1 cup sugar snap peas, red bell pepper, carrots, and/or other high-fiber veggies (page 345)

You'll Need: medium bowl, small bowl

Prep: 15 minutes

1. If you like, lightly toast bun halves/bread slices. Top each with a lettuce leaf and a tomato slice.

2. In a medium bowl, combine mayo, garlic powder, and onion powder. Add 1 tablespoon yogurt, and mix well. Add chicken, celery, and onion, and stir to coat.

3. Divide chicken mixture between bun halves/bread slices.

4. In a small bowl, mix ranch seasoning into remaining 2 tablespoons yogurt. Add 1 teaspoon water, and stir until uniform. Serve alongside sandwich, with veggies for dipping.

MAKES 1 SERVING

Grilled Veggie Sandwich
with side salad

Entire recipe: 330 calories, 8.5g fat, 607mg sodium, 40.5g carbs, 11g fiber, 11g sugars, 30g protein

SANDWICH

Half of a medium zucchini (cut widthwise), end removed

Half of a medium red bell pepper (cut lengthwise), stem and seeds removed

One 100-calorie flat sandwich bun

1 tablespoon hummus

1 tablespoon fat-free plain Greek yogurt

1 teaspoon chopped fresh basil

⅛ teaspoon garlic powder

SIDE SALAD

1 cup lettuce

¼ cup frozen shelled ready-to-eat edamame (unsalted), thawed

2 tablespoons crumbled reduced-fat feta cheese

3 chopped hard-boiled egg whites

2 teaspoons vinegar (balsamic, red wine, white wine, rice, or cider)

You'll Need: grill pan, nonstick spray, small bowl, medium bowl

Prep: 10 minutes

Cook: 10 minutes

Chill: 30 minutes (optional)

1. Slice both the zucchini half and the pepper half lengthwise into thirds.

2. Bring a grill pan sprayed with nonstick spray to medium-high heat. Grill veggies until softened and slightly blackened, about 5 minutes per side.

3. If you like, let cool completely; then cover and refrigerate veggies until chilled, at least 30 minutes.

4. If you like, lightly toast bun halves.

5. In a small bowl, combine hummus, yogurt, basil, and garlic powder. Mix well, and spread onto bun halves.

6. Blot away excess moisture from veggies, and layer them on the bottom bun half. Finish with the top bun half.

7. Toss salad ingredients in a medium bowl, and serve with sandwich.

MAKES 1 SERVING

BBQ Burger
with side salad 📷

Entire recipe: 348 calories, 8.5g fat, 556mg sodium, 38g carbs, 9g fiber, 11g sugars, 32.5g protein

BURGER

One 100-calorie flat sandwich bun

1 lettuce leaf

1 large tomato slice

4 ounces raw extra-lean ground beef (4% fat or less)

1 tablespoon egg whites or fat-free liquid egg substitute

⅛ teaspoon garlic powder

⅛ teaspoon onion powder

Dash each salt and black pepper

1 onion slice (rings intact)

1½ teaspoons BBQ sauce with 45 calories or less per 2-tablespoon serving

(continued on next page)

You'll Need: 2 medium bowls, grill pan (or skillet), nonstick spray

Prep: 15 minutes

Cook: 10 minutes

1. If you like, lightly toast bun halves. Top the bottom half with lettuce and tomato.

2. In a medium bowl, combine beef, egg whites/ substitute, and seasonings. Mix thoroughly. Evenly form into a 4-inch-wide patty.

3. Bring a grill pan (or skillet) sprayed with nonstick spray to medium-high heat. Cook patty for 3 to 4 minutes.

4. Flip patty, and add onion slice to the pan. Cook for 2 minutes.

5. Flip onion, and cook patty and onion until cooked to your preference, about 2 more minutes.

SIDE SALAD

1 cup lettuce

½ cup tomato, onion, and/or other high-fiber veggies (page 345)

½ cup cucumber, mushrooms, and/or other high-volume veggies (page 345)

2½ teaspoons vinegar (balsamic, red wine, white wine, rice, or cider)

½ teaspoon extra-virgin olive oil or grapeseed oil

6. Place patty on the bottom bun half. Top with onion and BBQ sauce, followed by the top bun.

7. Toss salad ingredients in a second medium bowl, and serve alongside your burger.

MAKES 1 SERVING

Sautéed Onion 'Bella Cheeseburger *with side salad*

Entire recipe: 344 calories, 8.5g fat, 630mg sodium, 43.5g carbs, 10.5g fiber, 12g sugars, 29.5g protein

BURGER

One 100-calorie flat sandwich bun

⅓ cup chopped onion

1 teaspoon Dijon mustard

1 teaspoon balsamic vinegar

Dash garlic powder

Dash cayenne pepper

1 portabella mushroom cap (stem removed)

1 slice Sargento Reduced Fat Swiss cheese

1 teaspoon light mayonnaise

(continued on next page)

You'll Need: skillet with a lid, nonstick spray, small bowl, medium bowl

Prep: 10 minutes

Cook: 10 minutes

1. If you like, lightly toast bun halves.

2. Bring a skillet sprayed with nonstick spray to medium-high heat. Cook and stir onion until softened and browned, about 2 minutes.

3. Transfer onion to a small bowl. Add mustard, balsamic vinegar, garlic powder, and cayenne pepper. Mix well, and cover to keep warm.

4. If needed, clean skillet. Re-spray, and return to medium-high heat. Add mushroom cap to the skillet, rounded side down. Cover and cook for 6 minutes, or until soft.

5. Flip mushroom, and top with cheese. Cook until cheese has melted, about 1 minute.

SIDE SALAD

2 cups lettuce

½ cup cucumber, mushrooms, and/or other high-volume veggies (page 345)

3 chopped hard-boiled egg whites

1 tablespoon crumbled reduced-fat feta cheese

2½ teaspoons vinegar (balsamic, red wine, white wine, rice, or cider)

6. Place mushroom cap on the bottom bun half, and top with onion mixture. Spread the top bun half with mayo, and place over the mushroom cap.

7. Toss salad ingredients in a medium bowl, and serve with your burger.

MAKES 1 SERVING

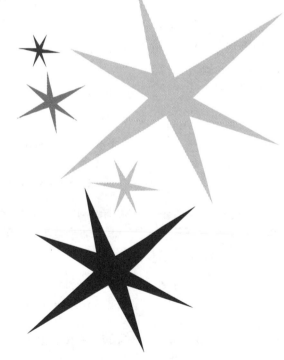

Caprese Portabella Burger
with side salad 📷

Entire recipe: 330 calories, 8g fat, 655mg sodium, 38g carbs, 10.5g fiber, 10g sugars, 31g protein

BURGER

One 100-calorie flat sandwich bun

2 tomato slices

1 portabella mushroom cap (stem removed)

⅛ teaspoon garlic powder

⅛ teaspoon onion powder

Dash black pepper

2 slices Sargento Reduced Fat Provolone cheese

1 tablespoon chopped basil

SIDE SALAD

2 cups lettuce

½ cup cucumber, mushrooms, or other high-volume veggies (page 345)

3 chopped hard-boiled egg whites

2½ teaspoons vinegar (balsamic, red wine, white wine, rice, or cider)

You'll Need: skillet with a lid, nonstick spray, medium bowl

Prep: 5 minutes

Cook: 10 minutes

1. If you like, lightly toast bun halves. Place tomato slices over the bottom half.

2. Bring a skillet sprayed with nonstick spray to medium-high heat. Place mushroom cap in the skillet, rounded side down. Cover and cook for 6 minutes, or until soft.

3. Flip mushroom, and season with garlic powder, onion powder, and pepper. Top with cheese. Cook until cheese has melted, about 1 minute.

4. Transfer cheese-topped mushroom to the bottom half of the bun. Top with basil and the top half of the bun.

5. Toss salad ingredients in a medium bowl, and serve alongside your burger.

MAKES 1 SERVING

Chinese Chicken Salad Wrap

Entire recipe: 349 calories, 8.5g fat, 703mg sodium, 38.5g carbs, 9.5g fiber, 11g sugars, 38g protein

⅔ cup bagged broccoli cole slaw, chopped

1 tablespoon low-fat sesame-ginger dressing

1 medium-large high-fiber flour tortilla with 110 calories or less

4 ounces cooked and chopped skinless chicken breast

¼ cup mandarin orange segments packed In juice, drained

2 tablespoons chopped scallions

¼ ounce (about 1 tablespoon) sliced almonds

You'll Need: medium bowl, microwave-safe plate

Prep: 10 minutes

Cook: 5 minutes or less

1. In a medium bowl, combine chopped broccoli slaw with dressing, and toss to coat.

2. Microwave tortilla on a microwave-safe plate for 10 seconds, or until warm.

3. Distribute slaw mixture across the middle of the tortilla, and top with remaining ingredients.

4. Wrap up tortilla by first folding in one side (to keep the filling from escaping), and then rolling it up from the bottom.

MAKES 1 SERVING

Lettuce Wraps & Lettuce Cups

LOVE sandwiches, but not big
on the starchy carbs from bread
and buns? Good news, Hungry!
Here's an entire chapter of lettuce-
wrapped deliciousness . . .

Lettuce-Wrapped Taco Burger
with carrot fries & dip 📷

Entire Recipe: 330 calories, 9g fat, 728mg sodium, 34g carbs, 11g fiber, 14.5g sugars, 29g protein

⅓ cup fat-free plain Greek yogurt

¼ teaspoon plus 1 dash ground cumin

¼ teaspoon plus 1 dash chili powder

7 ounces peeled carrots (about 1½ large carrots), cut into French-fry-shaped spears

1 frozen meatless hamburger-style patty with 100 calories or less

Dash garlic powder

Dash onion powder

¼ cup shredded reduced-fat Mexican-blend cheese

4 large (or 2 extra-large) iceberg or butter lettuce leaves

2 tablespoons chopped tomato

1 teaspoon chopped cilantro

You'll Need: baking sheet, nonstick spray, small bowl, skillet

Prep: 20 minutes

Cook: 25 minutes

1. Preheat oven to 400 degrees. Spray a baking sheet with nonstick spray.

2. In a small bowl, combine yogurt with ¼ teaspoon each cumin and chili powder. Mix well, and refrigerate until ready to serve.

3. Lay carrot spears on the baking sheet.

4. Bake for 15 minutes.

5. Flip spears. Bake until tender on the inside and slightly crispy on the outside, about 10 more minutes.

6. Meanwhile, bring a skillet sprayed with nonstick spray to medium heat. Cook patty for 4 minutes.

7. Flip patty, and sprinkle with garlic powder, onion powder, and remaining dash each cumin and chili powder. Top with cheese. Cook until cheese has melted and patty is cooked through, about 4 minutes.

8. Stack two large lettuce leaves, and place burger patty in the center (or stack two extra-large leaves, and place patty over one half). Top with half of the seasoned yogurt, followed by tomato and cilantro. Finish with the remaining two large lettuce leaves (or wrap the extra-large leaves around the filling).

9. Serve with carrot fries and remaining seasoned yogurt for dipping.

MAKES 1 SERVING

Lettuce-Wrapped Turkey Burger
with southwestern black beans

Entire recipe: 333 calories, 8.5g fat, 699mg sodium, 31.5g carbs, 7g fiber, 8g sugars, 33.5g protein

1 tablespoon fat-free plain Greek yogurt

2 teaspoons yellow mustard

2 teaspoons sweet relish

4 ounces raw lean ground turkey (7% fat or less)

1 tablespoon chopped onion

1 tablespoon egg whites or fat-free liquid egg substitute

⅛ teaspoon garlic powder

Dash black pepper

½ cup canned black beans, drained and rinsed

2 tablespoons salsa or pico de gallo with 90mg sodium or less per 2-tablespoon serving

4 large (or 2 extra-large) iceberg or butter lettuce leaves

1 large tomato slice

You'll Need: small bowl, medium bowl, grill pan (or skillet), nonstick spray, small microwave-safe bowl

Prep: 15 minutes

Cook: 15 minutes

1. To make the sauce, in a small bowl, combine yogurt, mustard, and relish. Mix well.

2. In a medium bowl, combine turkey, onion, egg whites/substitute, garlic powder, and pepper. Evenly form into a 4-inch-wide patty.

3. Bring a grill pan (or skillet) sprayed with nonstick spray to medium-high heat. Cook patty for 5 minutes per side, or until cooked through.

4. Meanwhile, combine black beans with salsa/pico de gallo in a small microwave-safe bowl. Cover and microwave for 1 minute, or until hot. Mix well.

5. Stack two large lettuce leaves, and place tomato in the center (or stack two extra-large leaves, and place tomato over one half). Top with turkey patty and sauce, and finish with the remaining two large lettuce leaves (or wrap the extra-large leaves around the filling).

6. Serve with black beans.

MAKES 1 SERVING

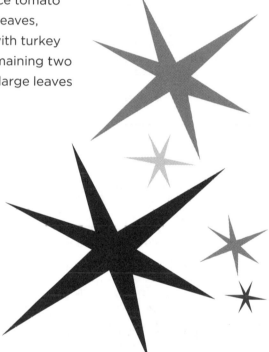

Lettuce-Wrapped Mushroom Swiss Burger *with carrot fries*

Entire recipe: 346 calories, 9.5g fat, 740mg sodium, 32.5g carbs, 8g fiber, 16.5g sugars, 35.5g protein

FRIES

8 ounces peeled carrots (about 1½ large carrots), cut into French-fry-shaped spears

Dash salt

1 tablespoon ketchup

BURGER

4 ounces raw extra-lean ground beef (4% fat or less)

Dash garlic powder

Dash onion powder

Dash each salt and black pepper

1 cup sliced brown mushrooms

1 slice Sargento Reduced Fat Swiss cheese

4 large (or 2 extra-large) iceberg or butter lettuce leaves

You'll Need: baking sheet, nonstick spray, medium bowl, grill pan (or large skillet)

Prep: 15 minutes

Cook: 25 minutes

1. Preheat oven to 400 degrees. Spray a baking sheet with nonstick spray.

2. Lay carrot spears on the sheet, and bake for 15 minutes.

3. Flip spears. Bake until tender on the inside and slightly crispy on the outside, about 10 minutes.

4. Meanwhile, in a medium bowl, combine beef with seasonings. Mix thoroughly, and form into a 4-inch patty.

5. Bring a grill pan (or large skillet) sprayed with nonstick spray to medium-high heat. Cook patty for 3 minutes.

6. Flip patty, and add mushrooms to the pan. Stirring mushrooms, cook for 3 to 4 more minutes, until patty is cooked to your preference and mushrooms have softened. Top patty with cheese, and cook until melted, about 1 minute.

7. Stack two large lettuce leaves, and place cheese-topped patty in the center (or stack two extra-large leaves, and place patty over one half). Top with mushrooms, and finish with the remaining two large lettuce leaves (or wrap the extra-large leaves around the filling).

8. Sprinkle fries with salt. Serve alongside burger, with ketchup for dipping.

MAKES 1 SERVING

For the latest food news, recipes, tips 'n tricks, and more, **sign up for free daily emails at hungry-girl.com!**

Cheesy Chicken Avocado Lettuce Wrap *with southwestern veggies*

Entire recipe: 337 calories, 9.5g fat, 581mg sodium, 28g carbs, 7g fiber, 8.5g sugars, 33g protein

One 4-ounce raw boneless skinless chicken breast cutlet, pounded to ½-inch thickness

2 dashes garlic powder

Dash each salt and black pepper

½ cup frozen sweet corn kernels

½ cup frozen broccoli florets

2 tablespoons southwestern salsa

4 large (or 2 extra-large) iceberg or butter lettuce leaves

1 tomato slice

1 wedge The Laughing Cow Light Creamy Swiss cheese

1 ounce thinly sliced avocado (about ¼ of an avocado)

You'll Need: skillet, nonstick spray, medium microwave-safe bowl

Prep: 10 minutes

Cook: 10 minutes

1. Bring a skillet sprayed with nonstick spray to medium heat. Add chicken, and sprinkle with seasonings. Cook for about 4 minutes per side, until cooked through.

2. Meanwhile, combine frozen veggies in a medium microwave-safe bowl. Cover and microwave for 1 minute and 30 seconds, or until hot. Add salsa, and mix well.

3. Stack two large lettuce leaves, and place tomato in the center (or stack two extra-large leaves, and place tomato over one half). Top with chicken, and spread with cheese wedge. Top with avocado, and finish with the remaining two large lettuce leaves (or wrap the extra-large leaves around the filling).

4. Serve with veggies.

MAKES 1 SERVING

Breakfasts

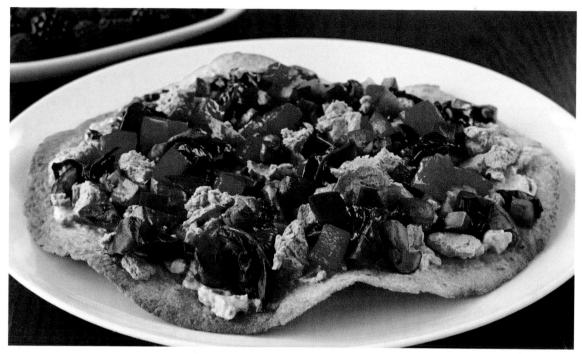

Guac 'n Veggie B-fast Tostada *with fruit* | p. 20

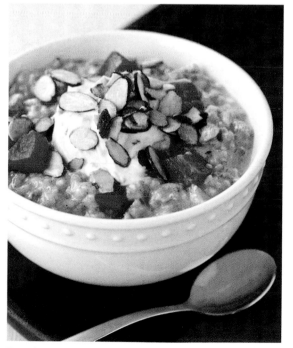

Peaches 'n Cream Oatmeal | p. 42

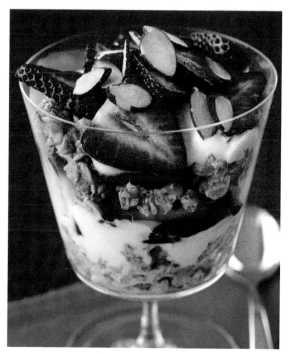

Overnight Oatmeal Parfait | p. 48

Breakfasts

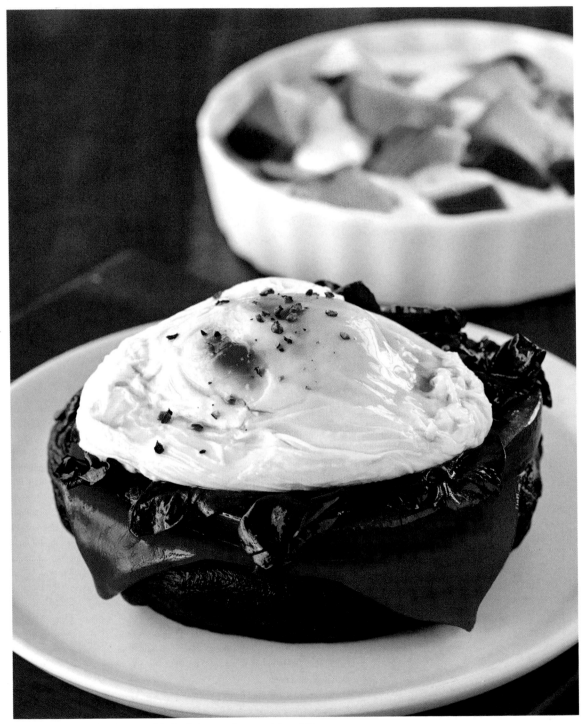

Portabella Poached Egg *with fruit-topped yogurt* | p. 36

Breakfasts

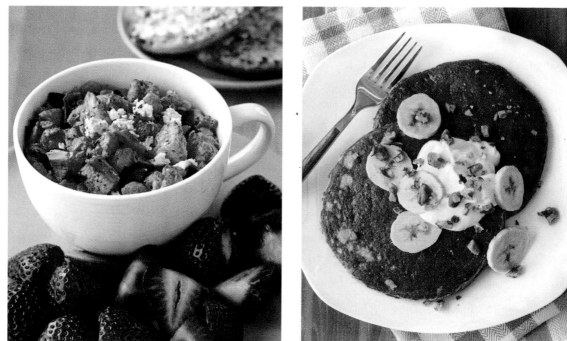

Chicken Feta Egg Mug *with bun and fruit* | p. 26

Banana Walnut Pancakes | p. 70

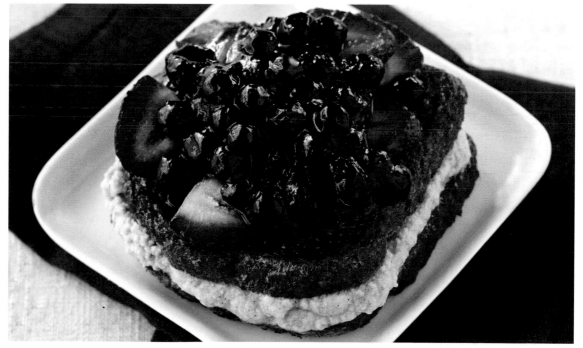

Stuffed 'n Smothered Berry French Toast | p. 76

Breakfasts

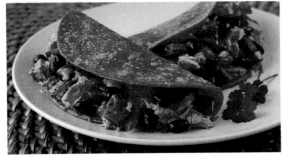

Breakfast Soft Tacos | p. 33

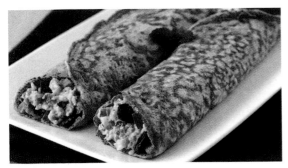

Apple Strudel Crepes | p. 82

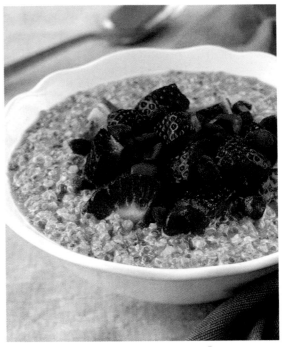

Strawberry Pistachio Quinoa | p. 51

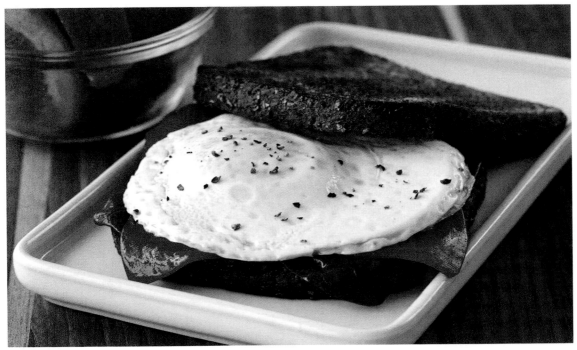

Over-Medium Egg Sandwich *with fruit* | p. 24

Lunches & Dinners

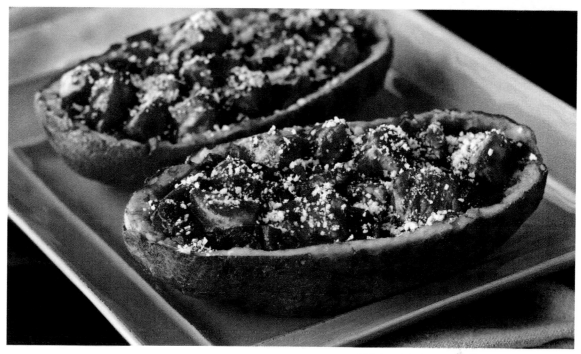

Chicken Marinara Stuffed Potato | p. 104

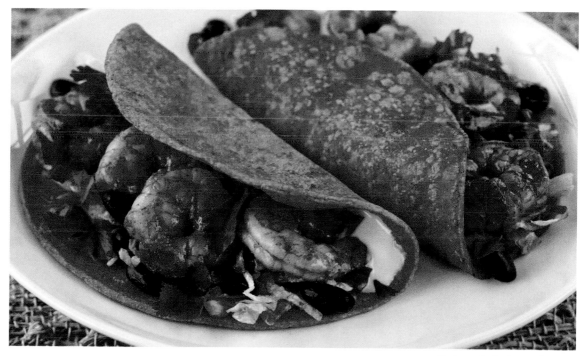

Shrimp Soft Tacos | p. 116

Lunches & Dinners

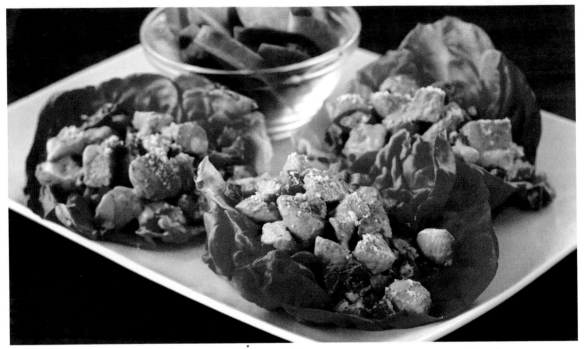

Buffalo Chicken Lettuce Cups *with apple slices* | p. 180

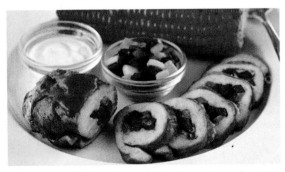

Southwest Chicken Bake *with buttered corn* | p. 222

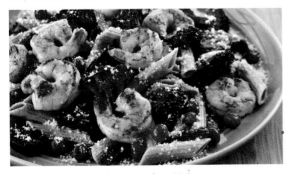

Shrimp & Pasta Primavera | p. 186

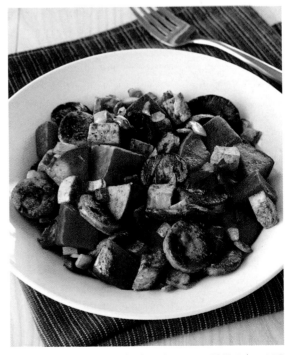

Butternut Squash & Chicken Sausage Skillet | p. 105

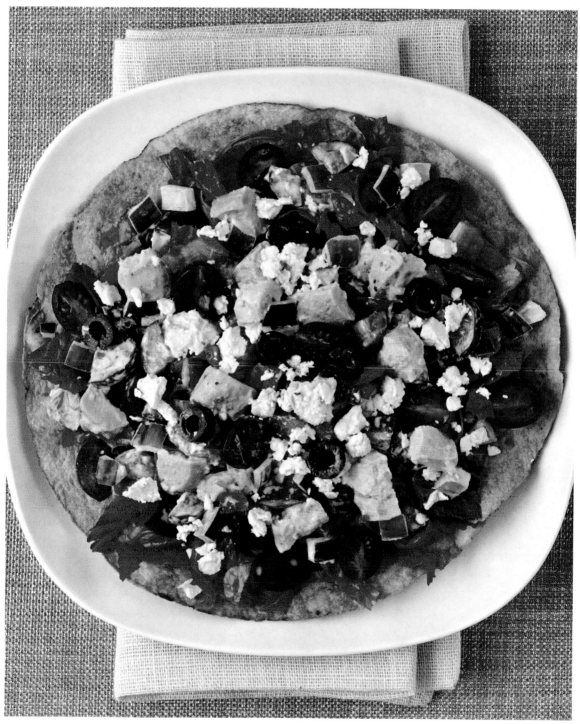

Greek Salad Tostada | p. 123

Lunches & Dinners

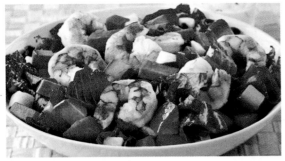

Tropical Shrimp Salad | p. 150

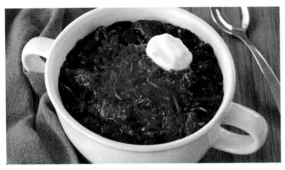

Chicken Chili | p. 134

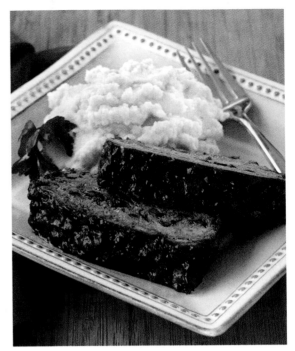

Meatloaf 'n Mashies | p. 226

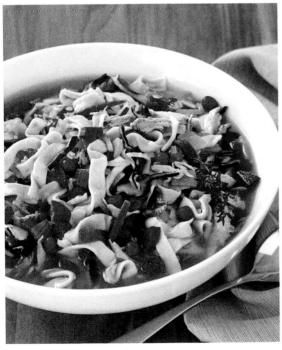

Chicken Noodle Bowl | p. 132

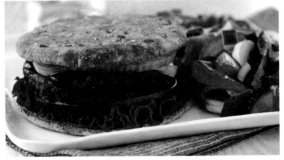

BBQ Burger *with side salad* | p. 158

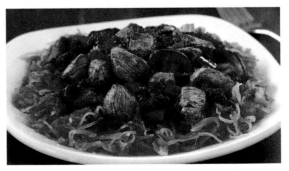

Chicken Cacciatore 'n Spaghetti Squash | p. 206

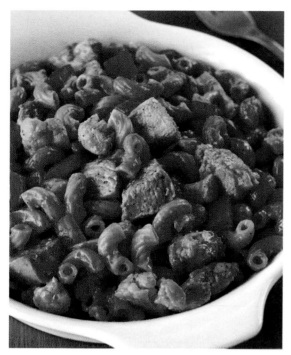

Mac 'n Chicken 'n Cheese | p. 184

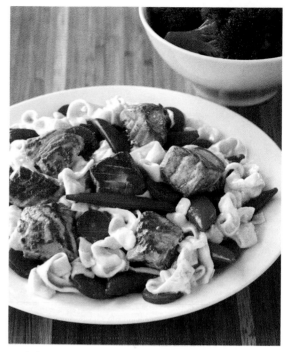

Salmon Girlfredo *with steamed broccoli* | p. 192

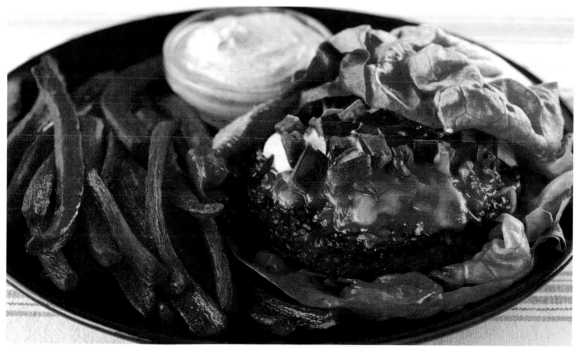

Lettuce-Wrapped Taco Burger *with carrot fries & dip* | p. 166

Lunches & Dinners

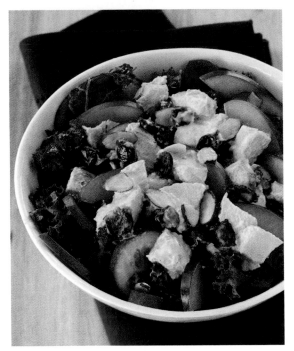

Cranberry Kale Chicken Salad | p. 147

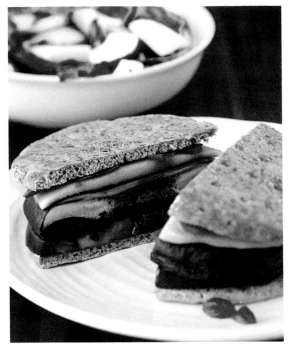

Caprese Portabella Burger *with side salad* | p. 162

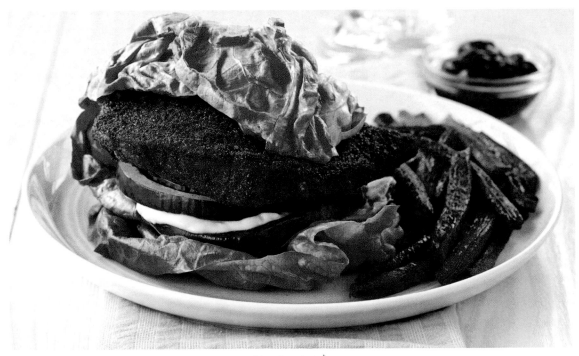

Lettuce-Wrapped Crispy Chicken *with carrot fries* | p. 174

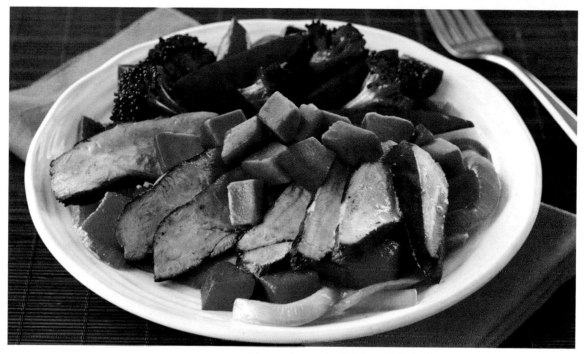

Mango Avocado Chicken Skillet *with steamed veggies* | p. 98

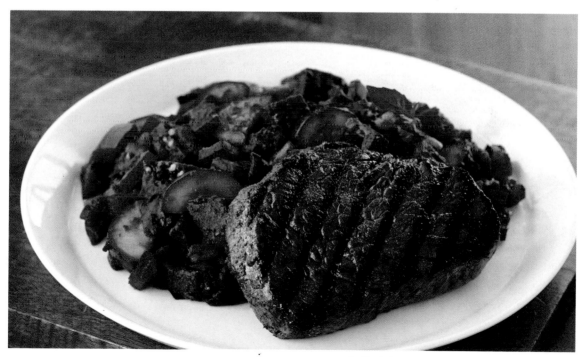

Grilled Steak with Ratatouille Pack | p. 214

Lunches & Dinners

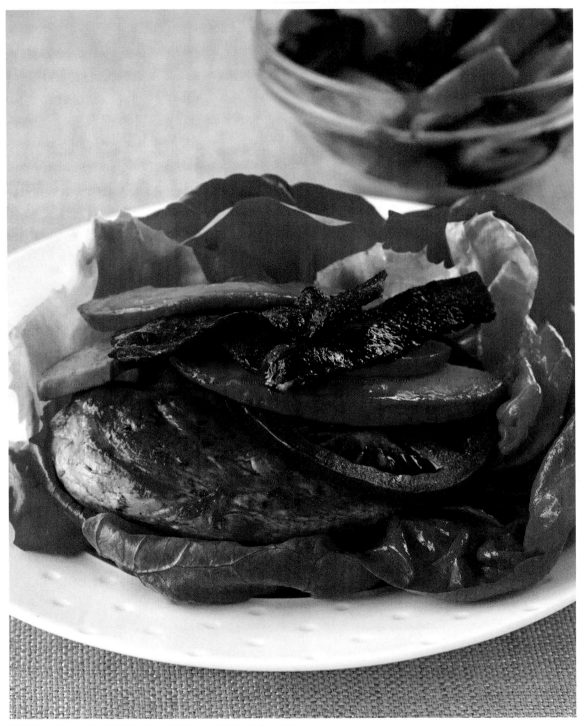

Chicken-Avocado BLT Lettuce Wrap *with fruit* | p. 176

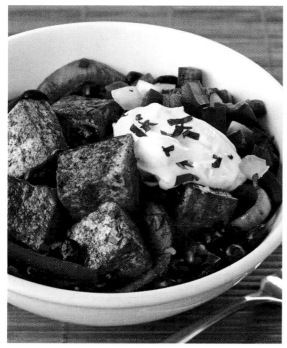

Fajita Tofu Bowl | p. 139

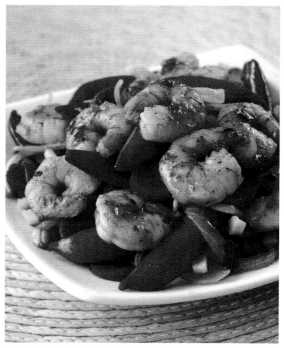

Sweet 'n Spicy Shrimp Stir-Fry | p. 94

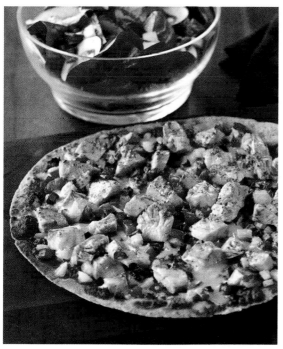

Chicken Veggie Pizza *with side salad* | p. 230

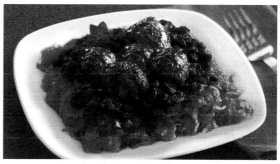

Spaghetti Squash with Meatballs | p. 208

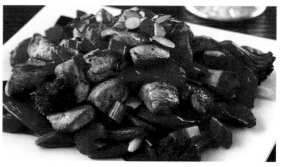

Chinese Chicken Stir-Fry | p. 90

Snacks

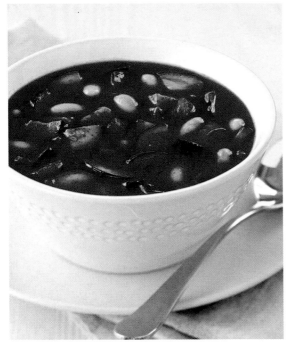

Pumpkin Veggie Soup | p. 259

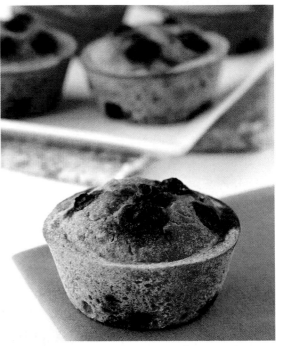

Blueberry Lemon Super Muffins | p. 299

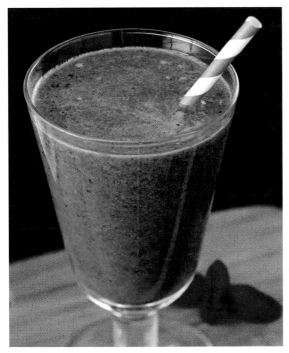

Peach-Berry Freeze | p. 274

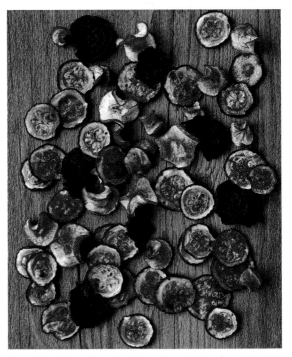

Zucchini Chips, Parsnip Chips, Beet Chips | p. 245–247

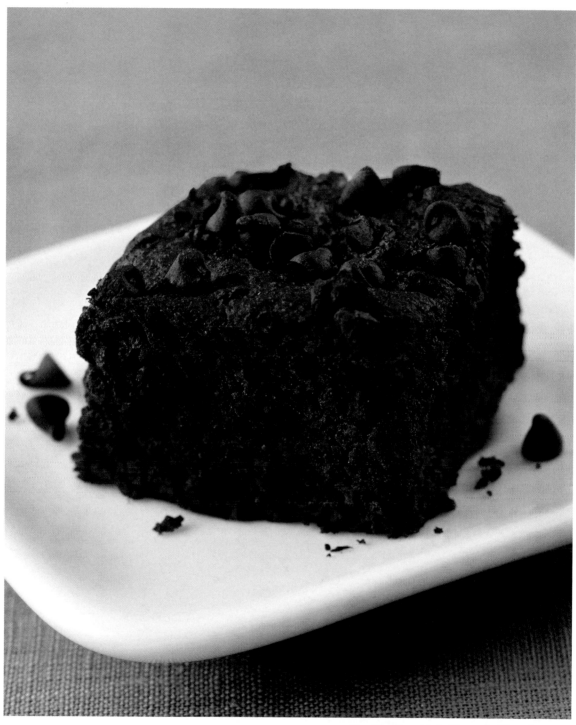

Double-Chocolate Brownie Bites | p. 297

Snacks

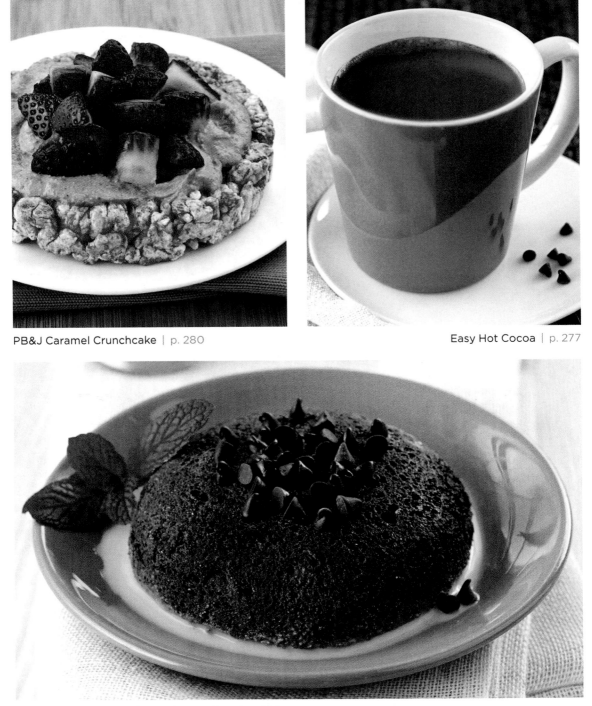

PB&J Caramel Crunchcake | p. 280

Easy Hot Cocoa | p. 277

Protein-Packed Chocolate Cake in a Mug | p. 298

Lettuce-Wrapped Roast Beef Sandwich *with veggies and tomato-ranch dip*

Entire recipe: 330 calories, 8g fat, 746mg sodium, 27.5g carbs, 8.5g fiber, 13g sugars, 36g protein

SANDWICH

4 large (or 2 extra-large) iceberg or butter lettuce leaves

2 large tomato slices

1 thin slice red onion

4 ounces (4 to 8 slices) no-salt-added roast beef

1 wedge The Laughing Cow Light Creamy Swiss Cheese

1 tablespoon Best Foods/ Hellman's Dijonnaise

VEGGIES AND DIP

¼ cup canned crushed tomatoes

½ teaspoon ranch dressing/dip seasoning mix

1¾ cups sugar snap peas, red bell pepper, carrots, and/or other high-fiber veggies (page 345)

You'll Need: medium bowl

Prep: 10 minutes

1. To make the sandwich, stack two large lettuce leaves, and place tomato and onion in the center (or stack two extra-large leaves, and place tomato and onion over one half). Top with roast beef, and spread with cheese wedge and Dijonnaise. Finish with the remaining two large lettuce leaves (or wrap the extra-large leaves around the filling).

2. To make the dip, in a medium bowl, stir ranch seasoning into crushed tomatoes. Serve alongside sandwich, with veggies for dipping.

MAKES 1 SERVING

Lettuce-Wrapped Crispy Chicken
with carrot fries 📷

Entire recipe: 339 calories, 9.5g fat, 672mg sodium, 34g carbs, 10g fiber, 14.5g sugars, 32.5g protein

FRIES

6 ounces peeled carrot (about 1 large carrot), cut into French-fry-shaped spears

1 teaspoon olive oil or grapeseed oil

Dash salt

1 tablespoon ketchup

(continued on next page)

You'll Need: baking sheet, nonstick spray, medium bowl, 2 wide bowls, large skillet

Prep: 25 minutes

Cook: 25 minutes

1. Preheat oven to 400 degrees. Spray a baking sheet with nonstick spray.

2. In a medium bowl, drizzle carrot spears with oil, and toss to coat.

3. Lay spears on the baking sheet, and bake for 15 minutes.

4. Flip spears. Bake until tender on the inside and slightly crispy on the outside, about 10 more minutes.

📷 Photo Alert!

The camera icon next to the recipe name means flip to the insert to see a photo of this recipe. Find full-color photos of ALL the recipes at hungry-girl.com/books.

SANDWICH

2 tablespoons Fiber One Original bran cereal, finely crushed

1 teaspoon salt-free seasoning mix

⅛ teaspoon garlic powder

⅛ teaspoon onion powder

2 tablespoons egg whites or fat-free liquid egg substitute

One 4-ounce raw boneless skinless chicken breast cutlet, pounded to ½-inch thickness

4 large (or 2 extra-large) iceberg or butter lettuce leaves

1 large tomato slice

2 teaspoons light mayonnaise

1 slice red onion

5. Meanwhile, in a wide bowl, combine crushed cereal with salt-free seasoning, garlic powder, and onion powder. Mix well.

6. Place egg whites/substitute in another wide bowl. Coat chicken with egg, shake to remove excess, and coat with crumbs.

7. Bring a large skillet sprayed with nonstick spray to medium heat. Cook chicken for about 5 minutes per side, until cooked through.

8. Stack two large lettuce leaves, and place tomato in the center (or stack two extra-large leaves, and place tomato over one half). Spread with mayo, and top with onion and chicken. Finish with the remaining two large lettuce leaves (or wrap the extra-large leaves around the filling).

9. Sprinkle fries with salt, and serve with ketchup for dipping.

MAKES 1 SERVING

Chicken-Avocado BLT Lettuce Wrap
with fruit 📷

Entire recipe: 335 calories, 10.5g fat, 365mg sodium, 32g carbs, 7.5g fiber, 20.5g sugars, 31.5g protein

1 slice center-cut bacon or turkey bacon

One 4-ounce raw boneless skinless chicken breast cutlet, pounded to ½-inch thickness

2 dashes garlic powder

Dash each salt and black pepper

4 large (or 2 extra-large) iceberg or butter lettuce leaves

1 large tomato slice

1 ounce thinly sliced avocado (about ¼ of an avocado)

1 cup halved strawberries or 50 calories' worth of another fruit (page 341)

⅔ cup chopped pineapple or 50 calories' worth of another fruit (page 341)

You'll Need: skillet, microwave-safe plate (optional), nonstick spray, medium bowl

Prep: 10 minutes

Cook: 15 minutes

1. Cook bacon until crispy, either in a skillet over medium heat or on a microwave-safe plate in the microwave. (See package for cook time.)

2. Bring a skillet sprayed with nonstick spray to medium heat. Sprinkle chicken with seasonings, and cook for about 4 minutes per side, until cooked through.

3. Stack two large lettuce leaves, and place chicken in the center (or stack two extra-large leaves, and place chicken over one half). Top with tomato and avocado. Break bacon in half, and place over avocado. Finish with the remaining two large lettuce leaves (or wrap the extra-large leaves around the filling).

4. Toss fruit in a medium bowl, and serve with wrap.

MAKES 1 SERVING

Asian Chicken Lettuce Cups

Entire recipe: 330 calories, 7.5g fat, 586mg sodium, 34g carbs, 5.5g fiber, 21g sugars, 34g protein

4 ounces cooked and chopped skinless chicken breast

1 cup peeled and diced cucumber

½ cup mandarin orange segments packed in juice, drained and roughly chopped

⅓ cup shredded carrot

¼ cup canned sliced water chestnuts, drained and roughly chopped

2 tablespoons chopped scallions

2 tablespoons low-fat sesame ginger dressing

⅛ teaspoon garlic powder

¼ ounce (about 1 tablespoon) sliced almonds

3 large iceberg or butter lettuce leaves

You'll Need: medium-large bowl

Prep: 10 minutes

1. In a medium-large bowl, combine all ingredients *except* lettuce leaves. Mix well.

2. Evenly distribute mixture among the lettuce leaves.

MAKES 1 SERVING

Need Chicken Cooking Tips?

Check out page 319, or purchase precooked chicken!

Tropical Shrimp Lettuce Cups

Entire recipe: 350 calories, 9.5g fat, 460mg sodium, 33.5g carbs, 9g fiber, 15.5g sugars, 36g protein

4½ ounces ready-to-eat shrimp (chopped, if large)

½ cup chopped mango

¼ cup chopped red onion

¼ cup canned black beans, drained and rinsed

1¾ ounces (about 3½ tablespoons) chopped avocado

2 tablespoons chopped cilantro

2 teaspoons lime juice

3 large iceberg or butter lettuce leaves

You'll Need: medium bowl

Prep: 10 minutes

---

1. In a medium bowl, combine all ingredients *except* lettuce leaves. Mix well.

2. Evenly distribute mixture among lettuce leaves.

MAKES 1 SERVING

Taco Lettuce Cups

Entire recipe: 345 calories, 8.5g fat, 651mg sodium, 32g carbs, 5.5g fiber, 12g sugars, 36.5g protein

4 ounces raw extra-lean ground beef (4% fat or less)

1 cup chopped brown mushrooms

½ cup chopped onion

1½ teaspoons taco seasoning mix

2 tablespoons frozen sweet corn kernels

2 tablespoons canned black beans, drained and rinsed

3 large iceberg or butter lettuce leaves

2 tablespoons shredded reduced-fat Mexican-blend cheese

½ cup chopped tomato

2 tablespoons fat-free plain Greek yogurt

2 tablespoons salsa or pico de gallo with 90mg sodium or less per 2-tablespoon serving

You'll Need: skillet, nonstick spray

Prep: 10 minutes

Cook: 10 minutes

1. Bring a skillet sprayed with nonstick spray to medium-high heat. Add beef, mushrooms, and onion. Cook, stir, and crumble until beef is fully cooked and veggies have softened, about 5 minutes.

2. Sprinkle with taco seasoning, and continue to cook until excess moisture has evaporated. Add corn and beans, and cook and stir until hot, about 1 minute.

3. Let cool slightly. Evenly distribute mixture among lettuce leaves. Top with cheese, tomato, yogurt, and salsa/pico de gallo.

MAKES 1 SERVING

Buffalo Chicken Lettuce Cups
with apple slices 📷

Entire recipe: 344 calories, 8.5g fat, 670mg sodium, 32.5g carbs, 7g fiber, 21.5g sugars, 34.5g protein

1½ teaspoons Frank's RedHot Original Cayenne Pepper Sauce

3 tablespoons light sour cream

4½ ounces raw boneless skinless chicken breast, cut into bite-sized pieces

⅛ teaspoon garlic powder

⅛ teaspoon onion powder

½ teaspoon ranch dressing/dip seasoning mix

⅔ cup chopped carrots

⅔ cup chopped celery

3 large iceberg or butter lettuce leaves

1 teaspoon grated Parmesan cheese

1 cup sliced apple

You'll Need: 2 medium bowls, skillet, nonstick spray

Prep: 10 minutes

Cook: 5 minutes

1. In a medium bowl, combine hot sauce with 1 tablespoon sour cream. Mix until uniform.

2. Bring a skillet sprayed with nonstick spray to medium-high heat. Add chicken, and sprinkle with garlic powder and onion powder. Cook and stir for about 4 minutes, until fully cooked.

3. Add chicken to the medium bowl, and stir to coat.

4. In another medium bowl, stir ranch mix into remaining 2 tablespoons sour cream. Add carrots and celery, and stir to coat.

5. Evenly distribute veggie mixture among the lettuce leaves, and top with saucy chicken and Parm.

6. Serve with apple slices.

MAKES 1 SERVING

Pineapple Steak Lettuce Cups

Entire recipe: 345 calories, 7g fat, 700mg sodium, 33.5g carbs, 4.5g fiber, 23g sugars, 39g protein

½ cup chopped onion

½ cup chopped bell pepper

5½ ounces raw lean beefsteak, cut into bite-sized pieces

Dash each salt and pepper

¼ cup canned crushed pineapple packed in juice

1 tablespoon sweet Asian chili sauce

1 teaspoon reduced-sodium/lite soy sauce

3 large iceberg or butter lettuce leaves

You'll Need: skillet, nonstick spray, medium bowl

Prep: 10 minutes

Cook: 10 minutes

1. Bring a skillet sprayed with nonstick spray to medium-high heat. Add onion and bell pepper. Cook and stir until slightly softened, about 3 minutes.

2. Add beef, and season with salt and black pepper. Cook until veggies have softened and beef is cooked through, about 3 minutes.

3. Transfer mixture to a medium bowl. Add pineapple, chili sauce, and soy sauce. Mix well.

4. Let cool slightly. Evenly distribute mixture among the lettuce cups.

MAKES 1 SERVING

Turkey BLT Lettuce Cups
with apple slices

Entire recipe: 337 calories, 9g fat, 690mg sodium, 33.5g carbs, 6.5g fiber, 23g sugars, 35.5g protein

3 slices center-cut bacon or turkey bacon

2 tablespoons fat-free plain Greek yogurt

¾ teaspoon ranch dressing/dip seasoning mix

3 ounces (3 to 6 slices) chopped no-salt-added turkey breast

3 large iceberg or butter lettuce leaves

¾ cup chopped tomato

1½ cups sliced apple

You'll Need: large skillet or microwave-safe plate, medium bowl

Prep: 10 minutes

Cook: 10 minutes

1. Cook bacon until crispy, either in a large skillet over medium heat or on a microwave-safe plate in the microwave. (See package for cook time.) Chop or crumble.

2. In a medium bowl, stir ranch mix into yogurt. Add chopped bacon and turkey, and stir to coat.

3. Evenly distribute mixture among the lettuce leaves, and top with tomatoes.

4. Serve with apple slices.

MAKES 1 SERVING

Hungry for More?

Don't miss the Mexi-Tuna Lettuce Cups on page 266!

Pasta & Pasta Swaps

Who doesn't love pasta?
These slimmed-down noodle
dishes and smart swaps are a hungry
girl's (or guy's!) BFF . . . Dig in!

Mac 'n Chicken 'n Cheese 📷

¼ of recipe (about 1¾ cups): 348 calories, 7g fat, 523mg sodium, 34g carbs, 6g fiber, 7g sugars, 36g protein

4½ ounces (about 1¼ cups) uncooked high-fiber elbow macaroni

3 cups frozen cauliflower florets

14 ounces raw boneless skinless chicken breast, cut into bite-sized pieces

¼ teaspoon garlic powder

¼ teaspoon onion powder

¼ teaspoon chili powder

¼ teaspoon each salt and black pepper

1 cup chopped yellow bell pepper

½ cup chopped onion

4 wedges The Laughing Cow Light Creamy Swiss cheese

2 tablespoons light sour cream

3 slices Sargento Reduced Fat Medium Cheddar cheese

You'll Need: medium-large pot, large microwave-safe bowl, large skillet, nonstick spray, small microwave-safe bowl

Prep: 15 minutes

Cook: 15 minutes

1. In a medium-large pot, cook pasta per package instructions, about 8 minutes.

2. Meanwhile, place cauliflower in a large microwave-safe bowl; cover and microwave for 3 minutes. Uncover and stir. Re-cover and microwave for 2 to 3 minutes, until cauliflower is hot. Drain excess liquid. Roughly chop cauliflower, and return to the bowl. Cover to keep warm.

3. Drain pasta, and add to the large bowl. Cover to keep warm.

4. Bring a large skillet sprayed with nonstick spray to medium-high heat. Add chicken, and sprinkle with ⅛ teaspoon of each seasoning. Add bell pepper and onion. Cook and stir for about 6 minutes, until chicken is fully cooked and veggies have softened and browned.

5. Add contents of the skillet to the large bowl. Re-cover to keep warm.

6. In a small microwave-safe bowl, stir cheese wedges until smooth. Add sour cream and cheese slices, breaking the slices into pieces. Add remaining ⅛ teaspoon of each seasoning. Mix well. Microwave for 1 minute. Stir mixture. Microwave for 30 seconds, or until hot and uniform.

7. Add cheese mixture to the large bowl. Stir until well mixed and thoroughly coated. If needed, microwave until hot.

MAKES 4 SERVINGS

Shrimp & Pasta Primavera 📷

¼ of recipe (about 2 cups): 339 calories, 8g fat, 648mg sodium, 34.5g carbs, 6.5g fiber, 6g sugars, 31.5g protein

4½ ounces (about 1¼ cups) uncooked high-fiber penne pasta

1½ cups chopped broccoli

1 cup thinly sliced red bell pepper cut into 1-inch pieces

½ cup chopped onion

1 pound (about 28) raw large shrimp, peeled, deveined, tails removed

1½ cups halved cherry tomatoes

½ cup frozen peas

¼ cup chopped fresh basil

1 tablespoon chopped garlic

1 tablespoon olive oil or grapeseed oil

¼ teaspoon each salt and black pepper

¼ cup grated Parmesan cheese

You'll Need: medium-large pot, large bowl, large skillet, nonstick spray

Prep: 15 minutes

Cook: 20 minutes

1. In a medium-large pot, cook pasta per package instructions, about 8 minutes.

2. Drain pasta, transfer to a large bowl, and cover to keep warm.

3. Meanwhile, bring a large skillet sprayed with nonstick spray to medium-high heat. Add broccoli, bell pepper, onion, and ⅓ cup water. Cover and cook until softened, about 6 minutes, uncovering occasionally to stir. Drain excess liquid, and transfer to the large bowl. Re-cover to keep warm.

4. Remove skillet from heat, re-spray, and return to medium-high heat. Add shrimp, tomatoes, and peas. Cook and stir for about 5 minutes, until shrimp are cooked through.

5. Add shrimp mixture to the large bowl, along with remaining ingredients *except* Parm. Mix well, and sprinkle with Parm.

MAKES 4 SERVINGS

Chicken Pesto Bowl

½ of recipe (about 2½ cups): 333 calories, 10.5g fat, 602mg sodium, 25.5g carbs, 10.5g fiber, 7g sugars, 40.5g protein

5 cups broccoli florets

2 bags House Foods Tofu Shirataki Spaghetti Shaped Noodle Substitute

¼ cup chopped fresh basil

½ cup light/low-fat ricotta cheese

1 tablespoon grated Parmesan cheese

2 teaspoons pine nuts

1 teaspoon chopped garlic

¼ teaspoon each salt and black pepper

8 ounces raw boneless skinless chicken breast, cut into bite-sized pieces

1½ teaspoons salt-free seasoning mix, or more to taste

You'll Need: large microwave-safe bowl, strainer, small blender or food processor, large skillet, nonstick spray

Prep: 15 minutes

Cook: 15 minutes

1. Place broccoli in a large microwave-safe bowl. Add ¼ cup water, cover, and microwave for 5 minutes, or until softened. Drain excess water, and re-cover to keep warm.

2. Use a strainer to rinse and drain noodles. Thoroughly pat dry. Roughly cut noodles.

3. To make the sauce, combine the following ingredients in a small blender or food processor: basil, ricotta cheese, Parmesan cheese, pine nuts, garlic, salt, and pepper. Add 3 tablespoons water. Blend until uniform.

4. Bring a large skillet sprayed with nonstick spray to medium-high heat. Add chicken, and sprinkle with ½ teaspoon salt-free seasoning. Cook and stir for about 4 minutes, until cooked through.

5. Reduce heat to medium. Add noodles, sauce, broccoli, and remaining 1 teaspoon salt-free seasoning. Cook and stir until hot and well mixed, about 2 minutes.

MAKES 2 SERVINGS

All About House Foods Tofu Shirataki

If you're unfamiliar with this pasta swap, listen up! These noodles are made of tofu and yam flour, resulting in a super-low-calorie alternative to traditional pasta. They've got JUST 20 CALORIES per two-serving bag, plus some fiber . . . and they're gluten-free!

Here are some things you need to know about Tofu Shirataki noodles . . .

1. They come floating in a bag of liquid . . . and they have a slight scent. Do not be alarmed! Just rinse and drain them well in a strainer.

2. Don't confuse these with plain shirataki noodles. Those are sometimes calorie-free, but the texture isn't as good. Tofu shirataki = way better.

3. Dry them. Well. Like *really* well. Grab a roll of paper towels, and start blotting! The more moisture you remove, the better your noodle dish will taste.

Find Tofu Shirataki in the refrigerated section of the supermarket, with the traditional tofu.

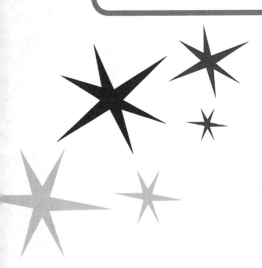

Mock Vodka Chicken Pasta

Entire recipe: 330 calories, 7g fat, 627mg sodium, 27g carbs, 9g fiber, 9g sugars, 39.5g protein

1 bag House Foods Tofu Shirataki Fettuccine Shaped Noodle Substitute

½ cup canned crushed tomatoes

⅛ teaspoon garlic powder

⅛ teaspoon onion powder

⅛ teaspoon black pepper

4½ ounces raw boneless skinless chicken breast, cut into bite-sized pieces

¼ teaspoon salt-free seasoning mix

1½ cups chopped brown mushrooms

⅓ cup frozen peas

2 tablespoons chopped fresh basil

1 wedge The Laughing Cow Light Original Swiss cheese

1½ teaspoons Parmesan cheese

You'll Need: strainer, small bowl, skillet, nonstick spray

Prep: 10 minutes

Cook: 10 minutes

1. Use a strainer to rinse and drain noodles. Thoroughly pat dry. Roughly cut noodles.

2. In a small bowl, combine crushed tomatoes, garlic powder, onion powder, and pepper. Mix well.

3. Bring a skillet sprayed with nonstick spray to medium-high heat. Add chicken, and sprinkle with salt-free seasoning. Add mushrooms. Cook and stir for about 4 minutes, until chicken is fully cooked and mushrooms have softened.

4. Reduce heat to medium. Add noodles, tomato mixture, peas, basil, and cheese wedge, breaking the wedge into pieces. Cook and stir until entire dish is hot and cheese has melted, mixed with tomatoes, and coated noodles, about 2 minutes.

5. Serve sprinkled with Parm.

MAKES 1 SERVING

Beef Stroganoff

Entire recipe: 344 calories, 9g fat, 740mg sodium, 32.5g carbs, 9.5g fiber, 9.5g sugars, 37g protein

1 bag House Foods Tofu Shirataki Fettuccine Shaped Noodle Substitute

4 ounces thinly sliced raw lean beefsteak

Dash each salt and black pepper

2 cups sliced mushrooms

1 cup chopped broccoli

¾ cup chopped onion

¼ cup fat-free or nearly fat-free beef gravy

1 wedge The Laughing Cow Light Creamy Swiss cheese

HG Tip!

Freeze your beef fillet slightly before cutting into it; this will make it easier to slice!

You'll Need: strainer, skillet with a lid, nonstick spray

Prep: 15 minutes

Cook: 15 minutes

1. Use a strainer to rinse and drain noodles. Thoroughly pat dry. Roughly cut noodles.

2. Bring a skillet sprayed with nonstick spray to medium-high heat. Add beef, and season with salt and pepper. Cook and stir for about 2 minutes, or until beef is just cooked through. Remove beef, and set aside.

3. Add mushrooms, broccoli, and onion to the skillet. Cover and cook for 5 minutes, or until soft. Uncover, and cook and stir until moisture has evaporated, about 1 minute.

4. Reduce heat to medium low. Add gravy and cheese wedge, breaking the wedge into pieces. Stir until cheese has melted and mixed with gravy, about 1 minute.

5. Add noodles and beef, and stir until completely coated and hot, about 2 minutes.

MAKES 1 SERVING

Shrimp Girlfredo
with steamed veggies

Entire recipe: 343 calories, 10.5g fat, 740mg sodium, 29g carbs, 12.5g fiber, 8.5g sugars, 35.5g protein

2 cups broccoli, cauliflower, Brussels sprouts, carrots, and/or asparagus

1 bag House Foods Tofu Shirataki Fettuccine Shaped Noodle Substitute

5 ounces (about 9) raw shrimp, peeled, tails removed, deveined

1 teaspoon olive oil or grapeseed oil

¼ teaspoon garlic powder

¼ teaspoon onion powder

1 tablespoon light sour cream

1 wedge The Laughing Cow Light Creamy Swiss cheese

You'll Need: medium microwave-safe bowl, strainer, skillet, nonstick spray

Prep: 10 minutes

Cook: 10 minutes

1. Place veggies in a medium microwave-safe bowl. Add 2 tablespoons water, cover, and microwave for 3 minutes, or until softened. Drain excess water, and re-cover to keep warm.

2. Meanwhile, use a strainer to rinse and drain noodles. Thoroughly pat dry. Roughly cut noodles.

3. Bring a skillet sprayed with nonstick spray to medium heat. Add shrimp, drizzle with oil, and sprinkle with ⅛ teaspoon of each seasoning. Cook and stir for about 3 minutes, until shrimp are cooked through.

4. To the skillet, add noodles, sour cream, and remaining ⅛ teaspoon of each seasoning. Add cheese wedge, breaking it into pieces. Cook and stir until cheese has melted, mixed with sour cream, and coated noodles, 2 to 3 minutes.

5. Top with steamed veggies (or serve veggies on the side).

MAKES 1 SERVING

Salmon Girlfredo
with steamed broccoli 📷

Entire recipe: 337 calories, 10g fat, 683mg sodium, 30.5g carbs, 13g fiber, 12g sugars, 29g protein

2½ cups broccoli florets

1 bag House Foods Tofu Shirataki Fettuccine Shaped Noodle Substitute

1 wedge The Laughing Cow Light Creamy Swiss cheese

⅛ teaspoon garlic powder, plus more to taste

⅛ teaspoon onion powder, plus more to taste

2 dashes each salt and black pepper

1 cup sugar snap peas

½ cup carrots sliced into coins

3 ounces raw skinless salmon fillet, cut into 1-inch cubes

1 tablespoon fat-free plain Greek yogurt

Optional seasoning: paprika

You'll Need: medium microwave-safe bowl, strainer, skillet, nonstick spray, medium bowl

Prep: 10 minutes

Cook: 10 minutes

1. Place broccoli in a medium microwave-safe bowl. Add 2 tablespoons water, cover, and microwave for 3 minutes, or until softened. Drain excess water, and re-cover to keep warm.

2. Meanwhile, use a strainer to rinse and drain noodles. Thoroughly pat dry. Roughly cut noodles.

3. Bring a skillet sprayed with nonstick spray to medium heat. Add noodles and cheese wedge, breaking the wedge into pieces. Cook and stir until cheese has melted and coated noodles, 2 to 3 minutes.

4. Transfer cheesy noodles to a medium bowl. Add garlic powder, onion powder, and a dash each salt and pepper. Mix well, and cover to keep warm.

5. Remove skillet from heat; clean, if needed. Re-spray, and bring to medium-high heat. Add snap peas and carrots.

6. Add salmon to the skillet, and season with remaining dash each salt and pepper. Stirring veggies and gently flipping salmon to evenly cook on all sides, cook until veggies have softened and browned and salmon is cooked through, about 4 minutes.

7. Stir yogurt into noodles, top noodles with contents of the skillet, and serve with steamed broccoli.

MAKES 1 SERVING

Thai Chicken Girlfredo

Entire recipe: 348 calories, 8.5g fat, 535mg sodium, 33.5g carbs, 11.5g fiber, 13g sugars, 37g protein

1 bag House Foods Tofu Shirataki Fettuccine Shaped Noodle Substitute

1½ cups small broccoli florets

½ cup chopped red bell pepper

¼ cup chopped onion

½ teaspoon chopped ginger

½ teaspoon chopped garlic

4 ounces raw boneless skinless chicken breast, cut into bite-sized pieces

¼ teaspoon salt-free seasoning mix

⅓ cup chopped scallions

1½ tablespoons low-fat Thai peanut salad dressing or sauce

1 wedge The Laughing Cow Light Creamy Swiss cheese

2 tablespoons fat-free plain Greek yogurt

You'll Need: strainer, skillet with a lid, nonstick spray, medium-large bowl

Prep: 10 minutes

Cook: 10 minutes

1. Use a strainer to rinse and drain noodles. Thoroughly pat dry. Roughly cut noodles.

2. Bring a skillet sprayed with nonstick spray to medium-high heat. Add broccoli, pepper, onion, ginger, garlic, and ¼ cup water. Cover and cook for 3 minutes, or until partially softened. Uncover, and cook and stir until water has evaporated and veggies have softened, about 2 minutes. Transfer to a medium-large bowl, and cover to keep warm.

3. Remove skillet from heat; clean, if needed. Re-spray, and return to medium-high heat. Add chicken, and sprinkle with salt-free seasoning. Cook and stir for about 4 minutes, until cooked through.

4. Reduce heat to medium. Add noodles, scallions, dressing/sauce, and cheese wedge, breaking the wedge into pieces. Cook and stir until cheese has melted, mixed with dressing/sauce, and coated noodles, about 1 minute.

5. Transfer contents of the skillet to the bowl. Add yogurt, and mix well.

MAKES 1 SERVING

Southwest Chicken Girlfredo

Entire recipe: 349 calories, 10g fat, 554mg sodium, 30.5g carbs, 8.5g fiber, 7.5g sugars, 34.5g protein

1 bag House Foods Tofu Shirataki Fettuccine Shaped Noodle Substitute

¼ cup chopped bell pepper

4 ounces raw boneless skinless chicken breast, cut into bite-sized pieces

½ teaspoon salt-free seasoning mix

¼ cup frozen sweet corn kernels

3 tablespoons light sour cream

¼ cup canned black beans, drained and rinsed

½ teaspoon taco seasoning mix

1 wedge The Laughing Cow Light Creamy Swiss cheese

You'll Need: strainer, skillet, nonstick spray

Prep: 10 minutes

Cook: 10 minutes

1. Use a strainer to rinse and drain noodles. Thoroughly pat dry. Roughly cut noodles.

2. Bring a skillet sprayed with nonstick spray to medium-high heat. Cook pepper until slightly softened, about 2 minutes.

3. Add chicken to the skillet, and sprinkle with salt-free seasoning. Add corn, and cook and stir until pepper has softened and slightly browned, chicken is fully cooked, and corn is hot, about 4 minutes.

4. Reduce heat to medium. Add remaining ingredients, breaking the cheese wedge into pieces. Cook and stir until cheese has melted, mixed with sour cream, and coated noodles, 2 to 3 minutes.

MAKES 1 SERVING

Pumpkin Feta Chicken Girlfredo

Entire recipe: 350 calories, 10g fat, 617mg sodium, 28g carbs, 9g fiber, 9g sugars, 38.5g protein

1 bag House Foods Tofu Shirataki Fettuccine Shaped Noodle Substitute

¼ cup canned pure pumpkin

¼ cup fat-free milk

¼ teaspoon garlic powder

¼ teaspoon onion powder

Dash black pepper

2 cups chopped kale leaves

¼ cup chopped onion

¼ cup low-sodium chicken broth

½ teaspoon chopped garlic

4 ounces raw boneless skinless chicken breast, cut into bite-sized pieces

¼ teaspoon salt-free seasoning mix

1 wedge The Laughing Cow Light Creamy Swiss cheese

3 tablespoons crumbled reduced-fat feta cheese

You'll Need: strainer, medium bowl, skillet, nonstick spray, medium-large bowl

Prep: 15 minutes

Cook: 10 minutes

1. Use a strainer to rinse and drain noodles. Thoroughly pat dry. Roughly cut noodles.

2. In a medium bowl, combine pumpkin, milk, garlic powder, onion powder, and pepper. Mix until uniform.

3. Bring a skillet sprayed with nonstick spray to medium-high heat. Add kale, onion, chicken broth, and chopped garlic. Cook and stir until veggies have softened and broth has evaporated, about 3 minutes. Transfer to a medium-large bowl, and cover to keep warm.

4. Remove skillet from heat; clean, if needed. Re-spray, and return to medium-high heat. Add chicken, and sprinkle with salt-free seasoning. Cook and stir for about 4 minutes, until cooked through.

5. Reduce heat to medium. Add noodles, kale mixture, pumpkin mixture, and cheese wedge, breaking the wedge into pieces. Cook and stir until entire dish is hot and cheese has melted, mixed with pumpkin mixture, and coated noodles, about 2 minutes.

6. Serve topped with feta cheese.

MAKES 1 SERVING

Chicken Pad Thai
with cucumber salad

Entire recipe: 350 calories, 7.5g fat, 500mg sodium, 40g carbs, 9.5g fiber, 20g sugars, 36.5g protein

SALAD

1 tablespoon plain rice vinegar

½ teaspoon granulated white sugar

1 cup thinly sliced cucumber

¼ cup thinly sliced red onion

PAD THAI

1 bag House Foods Tofu Shirataki Fettuccine Shaped Noodle Substitute

1 tablespoon ketchup

1 tablespoon lime juice

½ tablespoon low-sugar apricot preserves

1 teaspoon brown sugar (not packed)

½ teaspoon reduced-sodium/lite soy sauce

¼ teaspoon chopped garlic

⅛ teaspoon crushed red pepper, or more to taste

(continued on next page)

You'll Need: medium bowl, whisk, strainer, small bowl, large skillet, nonstick spray, medium-large bowl

Prep: 20 minutes

Cook: 10 minutes

1. To make the salad, in a medium bowl, combine vinegar with sugar, and whisk to dissolve. Add cucumber and onion, and toss to coat. Cover and refrigerate until ready to serve.

2. Use a strainer to rinse and drain noodles. Thoroughly pat dry. Roughly cut noodles.

3. To make the sauce, in a small bowl, combine ketchup, lime juice, preserves, brown sugar, soy sauce, garlic, and crushed red pepper. Mix until uniform.

¼ cup fat-free liquid egg substitute

¾ cup chopped broccoli

¾ cup bean sprouts

3½ ounces raw boneless skinless chicken breast, cut into bite-sized pieces

¼ teaspoon salt-free seasoning mix

¼ cup 1-inch scallion pieces

¼ ounce (about 2½ teaspoons) crushed dry-roasted peanuts

1 tablespoon chopped cilantro

4. Bring a large skillet sprayed with nonstick spray to medium-high heat. Scramble egg substitute until fully cooked, about 1 minute. Transfer to a medium-large bowl, and cover to keep warm.

5. Remove skillet from heat; clean, if needed. Re-spray, and return to medium-high heat. Add broccoli, bean sprouts, and 2 tablespoons water. Cook and stir until water has evaporated and veggies have slightly softened, about 2 minutes.

6. Add chicken to the skillet, and sprinkle with salt-free seasoning. Cook and stir until veggies have softened and chicken is fully cooked, about 4 minutes.

7. Add noodles, sauce, scallions, and peanuts. Cook and stir until well mixed. Gently stir in scrambled egg substitute, and cook until hot, 1 to 2 minutes.

8. Transfer to the bowl, top with cilantro, and serve alongside salad.

MAKES 1 SERVING

Deconstructed Lasagna

Entire recipe: 344 calories, 9.5g fat, 750mg sodium, 38g carbs, 12g fiber, 18g sugars, 30.5g protein

1 bag House Foods Shirataki Spaghetti Shaped Noodle Substitute

3 ounces raw extra-lean ground beef (4% fat or less)

⅛ teaspoon Italian seasoning

⅛ teaspoon onion powder

1½ cups chopped broccoli

½ cup sliced mushrooms

½ cup chopped zucchini

¼ cup chopped onion

½ teaspoon chopped garlic

⅔ cup low-fat marinara sauce

2 tablespoons light/low-fat ricotta cheese

1 teaspoon grated Parmesan cheese

Optional seasoning: red pepper flakes

You'll Need: strainer, skillet, nonstick spray, medium bowl

Prep: 10 minutes

Cook: 15 minutes

1. Use a strainer to rinse and drain noodles. Thoroughly pat dry. Roughly cut noodles.

2. Bring a skillet sprayed with nonstick spray to medium-high heat. Add beef, and sprinkle with Italian seasoning and onion powder. Cook and crumble for about 3 minutes, until fully cooked. Transfer to a medium bowl, and cover to keep warm.

3. Remove skillet from heat; clean, if needed. Re-spray, and return to medium-high heat. Add all veggies, garlic, and ¼ cup water. Cook and stir until water has evaporated and veggies have softened, about 5 minutes.

4. Add noodles, beef, and marinara sauce. Cook and stir until hot and well mixed, 1 to 2 minutes.

5. Remove from heat, add ricotta, and mix thoroughly. Serve sprinkled with Parm.

MAKES 1 SERVING

Saucy Shrimp Marinara

Entire recipe: 336 calories, 8g fat, 709mg sodium, 35.5g carbs, 16g fiber, 15.5g sugars, 31.5g protein

4 cups bagged broccoli cole slaw

4 ounces (about 7) raw large shrimp, peeled, tails removed, deveined

1½ teaspoons olive oil or grapeseed oil

½ cup canned crushed tomatoes, drained

½ cup canned no-salt-added diced tomatoes, drained

¼ teaspoon garlic powder

¼ teaspoon onion powder

⅛ teaspoon black pepper

You'll Need: large skillet with a lid, nonstick spray, large bowl

Prep: 5 minutes

Cook: 15 minutes

1. Bring a large skillet sprayed with nonstick spray to medium-high heat. Add broccoli slaw and ½ cup water. Cover and cook for 8 minutes, or until fully softened. Uncover and, if needed, cook and stir until water has evaporated, 1 to 2 minutes. Transfer to a large bowl, and cover to keep warm.

2. Remove skillet from heat, re-spray, and bring to medium heat. Add shrimp, and drizzle with oil. Cook and stir for about 2 minutes, until shrimp are just cooked through.

3. To the skillet, add slaw, crushed tomatoes, diced tomatoes, and seasonings. Cook and stir until hot and well mixed, about 2 minutes.

MAKES 1 SERVING

Spaghetti Squash Chicken Girlfredo

¼ of recipe (about 2 cups): 337 calories, 7g fat, 630mg sodium, 28g carbs, 6.5g fiber, 12g sugars, 36g protein

1 spaghetti squash (at least 4½ pounds)

1 pound raw boneless skinless chicken breast, cut into bite-sized pieces

¼ teaspoon each salt and black pepper

2 cups sliced mushrooms

1 cup chopped onion

2 cups frozen peas

1½ teaspoons chopped garlic

2 tablespoons grated Parmesan cheese

6 wedges The Laughing Cow Light Creamy Swiss cheese

You'll Need: large baking pan, large skillet, nonstick spray, medium bowl, strainer, large bowl

Prep: 20 minutes

Cook: 55 minutes

1. Preheat oven to 400 degrees.

2. Microwave squash for 6 minutes, or until soft enough to cut. Once cool enough to handle, halve lengthwise; scoop out and discard seeds.

3. Fill a large baking pan with ½ inch water and place squash halves in the pan, cut sides down. Bake until tender, about 40 minutes.

4. Meanwhile, bring a large skillet sprayed with nonstick spray to medium-high heat. Add chicken, and season with ⅛ teaspoon each salt and pepper. Cook and stir for about 7 minutes, until cooked through. Transfer to a medium bowl, and cover to keep warm.

5. Use a fork to scrape out spaghetti squash strands. Place in a strainer to drain excess moisture. Thoroughly blot dry, removing as much moisture as possible. Transfer 5 cups to a large bowl. (Reserve any extra squash for another time.) Cover to keep warm.

6. If needed, clean skillet. Re-spray, and return to medium-high heat. Add mushrooms and onion. Cook and stir until mostly softened and slightly browned, 4 to 5 minutes. Add peas and garlic, and cook and stir until hot, about 2 minutes.

7. Reduce heat to low. Add Parmesan cheese and cheese wedges, breaking the wedges into pieces. Cook and stir until cheese has melted and coated veggies, about 2 minutes.

8. Add cheesy veggies to the large bowl. Add remaining ⅛ teaspoon each salt and pepper, and mix well. Top with chicken.

MAKES 4 SERVINGS

Spaghetti Squash Bolognese

¼ of recipe (about 2 cups): 330 calories, 8.5g fat, 717mg sodium, 33.5g carbs, 8g fiber, 15g sugars, 29.5g protein

1 spaghetti squash (at least 4½ pounds)

3½ cups canned crushed tomatoes

¼ cup tomato paste

1 tablespoon white wine vinegar

1 teaspoon Italian seasoning

1 teaspoon garlic powder

1 teaspoon onion powder

½ cup chopped celery

⅓ cup chopped onion

⅓ cup chopped carrots

1 tablespoon olive oil or grapeseed oil

1 pound raw extra-lean ground beef (4% fat or less)

¼ teaspoon salt

⅛ teaspoon black pepper

You'll Need: large baking pan, large bowl, large skillet, nonstick spray, strainer

Prep: 20 minutes

Cook: 50 minutes

1. Preheat oven to 400 degrees.

2. Microwave squash for 6 minutes, or until soft enough to cut. Once cool enough to handle, halve lengthwise; scoop out and discard seeds.

3. Fill a large baking pan with ½ inch water and place squash halves in the pan, cut sides down. Bake until tender, about 40 minutes.

4. Meanwhile, in a large bowl, combine crushed tomatoes, tomato paste, vinegar, and Italian seasoning. Add ½ teaspoon each garlic powder and onion powder, and mix well.

5. Bring a large skillet sprayed with nonstick spray to medium-high heat. Add celery, onion, and carrots, and drizzle with oil. Cook and stir until slightly softened, about 2 minutes.

6. Add beef to the skillet. Sprinkle with salt, pepper, and remaining ½ teaspoon each garlic powder and onion powder. Cook, stir, and crumble until veggies have softened and beef is fully cooked, about 8 minutes.

7. Carefully add tomato mixture to the skillet. Cook and stir until hot and well mixed, about 2 minutes. Remove from heat.

8. Use a fork to scrape out spaghetti squash strands. Place in a strainer to drain excess moisture. Thoroughly blot dry, removing as much moisture as possible. Transfer 5 cups to a large bowl. (Reserve any extra squash for another time.)

9. Top squash with saucy beef, stir, and serve.

MAKES 4 SERVINGS

Time-Saving Alternative: Cook Your Spaghetti Squash in the Microwave

Instead of baking the squash, try this! After scooping out and discarding the seeds, place one half of the squash in an extra-large microwave-safe bowl, cut side down. Add ¼ cup water, cover, and cook for 7 minutes, or until soft. Repeat with remaining squash half.

Chicken Cacciatore 'n Spaghetti Squash 📷

¼ of recipe (1¼ cups squash with about 1¼ cups veggie-chicken mixture and 1 tablespoon Parm): 330 calories, 7.5g fat, 693mg sodium, 31.5g carbs, 8g fiber, 14g sugars, 35g protein

1 spaghetti squash (at least 4½ pounds)

1 pound raw boneless skinless chicken breast, cut into bite-sized pieces

¼ teaspoon each salt and black pepper

2 cups chopped green bell pepper

2 cups sliced mushrooms

¾ cup chopped onion

1 teaspoon olive oil or grapeseed oil

2½ cups canned crushed tomatoes

1 teaspoon chopped garlic

½ teaspoon dried oregano

½ teaspoon dried basil

¼ teaspoon red pepper flakes

¼ teaspoon garlic powder

¼ teaspoon onion powder

¼ cup grated Parmesan cheese

You'll Need: large baking pan, large pot, nonstick spray, strainer, large bowl

Prep: 25 minutes

Cook: 50 minutes

1. Preheat oven to 400 degrees.

2. Microwave squash for 6 minutes, or until soft enough to cut. Halve lengthwise; scoop out and discard seeds.

3. Fill a large baking pan with ½ inch water and place squash halves in the pan, cut sides down. Bake until tender, about 40 minutes.

4. Meanwhile, bring a large pot sprayed with nonstick spray to medium-high heat. Add chicken, and season with salt and black pepper. Cook and stir for 3 minutes.

5. Add bell pepper, mushrooms, and onion to the pot. Drizzle with oil. Cook and stir for about 10 minutes, until chicken is fully cooked and veggies have softened.

6. Add crushed tomatoes to the pot, along with chopped garlic, oregano, basil, and red pepper flakes. Cook and stir until hot, about 2 minutes. Remove from heat and cover to keep warm.

7. Use a fork to scrape out spaghetti squash strands. Place in a strainer to drain excess moisture. Thoroughly blot dry, removing as much moisture as possible. Transfer 5 cups to a large bowl. (Reserve any extra squash for another time.) Add garlic powder and onion powder, and mix well.

8. Top each serving of squash (1¼ cups) with ¼ of chicken-veggie mixture (about 1¼ cups), and sprinkle with 1 tablespoon Parm.

MAKES 4 SERVINGS

Leftover Squash Idea!

Did your spaghetti squash yield more than 5 cups? (It happens.) Enjoy 1½ cups cooked squash with ¼ cup low-fat marinara sauce as a 100-calorie snack.

Spaghetti Squash with Meatballs 📷

¼ of recipe (1¼ cups squash with 5 meatballs and ¼ of the sauce): 346 calories, 6.5g fat, 701mg sodium, 32.5g carbs, 7.5g fiber, 14.5g sugars, 39g protein

SQUASH

1 spaghetti squash (at least 4½ pounds)

MEATBALLS

1¼ pounds raw extra-lean ground beef (4% fat or less)

½ cup egg whites or fat-free liquid egg substitute

1 teaspoon Italian seasoning

¼ teaspoon garlic powder

¼ teaspoon onion powder

⅛ teaspoon each salt and black pepper

(continued on next page)

You'll Need: baking sheet, nonstick spray, large baking pan, 2 large bowls, large pot with a lid, strainer

Prep: 30 minutes

Cook: 1 hour

1. Preheat oven to 400 degrees. Spray a baking sheet with nonstick spray.

2. Microwave squash for 6 minutes, or until soft enough to cut. Halve lengthwise; scoop out and discard seeds.

3. Fill a large baking pan with ½ inch water and place squash halves in the pan, cut sides down. Bake until tender, about 40 minutes.

4. Meanwhile, combine meatball ingredients in a large bowl, and mix thoroughly. (The mixture may be a little sticky—this is okay!) Firmly form into 20 evenly sized meatballs, and place on the baking sheet. Bake until just cooked through, about 10 minutes. (Meatballs can bake simultaneously with squash.)

SAUCE

3 cups finely chopped
mushrooms

1 cup chopped onion

3 cups canned crushed
tomatoes

1 tablespoon tomato paste

2 teaspoons Italian
seasoning

¼ teaspoon garlic powder

¼ teaspoon onion powder

⅛ teaspoon each salt and
black pepper

5. Bring a large pot sprayed with nonstick spray to medium-high heat. Add mushrooms and onion. Cook and stir until softened and browned, about 10 minutes. Reduce heat to low. Add remaining sauce ingredients, and mix well. Add meatballs, and cook and stir until hot, about 3 minutes. Remove from heat, and cover to keep warm.

6. Use a fork to scrape out spaghetti squash strands. Place in a strainer to drain excess moisture. Thoroughly blot dry, removing as much moisture as possible. Transfer 5 cups to a large bowl. (Reserve any extra squash for another time.)

7. Top each serving of squash (1¼ cups) with 5 meatballs and ¼ of the sauce.

MAKES 4 SERVINGS

Foil Packs & HG Bakes

Hungry Girl foil packs are mega popular, and with good reason: They cook quickly, and cleanup's a breeze! "HG Bakes" refers to anything made in the oven, and we've got some goodies here, from fish 'n chips to meatloaf 'n mashies!

Foil Pack 101

What's a foil pack? It's an easy-cleanup meal cooked in a DIY pouch of foil! Here are a few tips for foil-pack perfection . . .

- Heavy-duty aluminum foil is a must. No flimsy foil allowed!

- Don't skimp on the size of those foil sheets. Large ones are needed to allow for room above the food for steaming action!

- When you fold that foil, really seal those seams tightly—don't let the heat out.

- Why do all HG foil-pack recipes end with "Cut packet to release steam before opening entirely"? Because that steam is hot! Cutting a vent in the foil will allow the steam to escape safely.

- Having trouble with the cook times? Pick up an oven thermometer to check the temp inside your oven. You might be surprised to find that the built-in temperature gauge is off.

Apricot Chicken Pack

Entire recipe: 350 calories, 9g fat, 550mg sodium, 30g carbs, 6g fiber, 14g sugars, 38g protein

2 teaspoons cider vinegar

1 teaspoon cornstarch

1 teaspoon onion soup/dip seasoning mix

2 tablespoons low-sugar apricot preserves

2½ teaspoons light whipped butter or light buttery spread, room temperature

5 ounces raw boneless skinless chicken breast, cut into 1-inch cubes

Dash each salt and black pepper

2½ cups small broccoli florets

You'll Need: heavy-duty aluminum foil, baking sheet, nonstick spray, medium-large bowl, whisk

Prep: 10 minutes

Cook: 20 minutes

1. Preheat oven to 375 degrees. Lay a large piece of heavy-duty foil on a baking sheet, and spray with nonstick spray.

2. In a medium-large bowl, combine vinegar, cornstarch, and onion seasoning mix. Whisk to dissolve. Add preserves and butter, and whisk until mostly uniform.

3. Season chicken with salt and pepper, and add to the bowl. Add broccoli, and stir to coat. Distribute mixture onto the center of the foil.

4. Cover with another large piece of foil. Fold together and seal all four edges of the foil pieces, forming a well-sealed packet. Bake for 20 minutes, or until chicken is cooked through and broccoli is tender.

5. Cut packet to release steam before opening entirely.

MAKES 1 SERVING

Grilled Steak with Ratatouille Pack 📷

Entire recipe: 347 calories, 6.5g fat, 600mg sodium, 35.5g carbs, 9g fiber, 18.5g sugars, 39.5g protein

½ cup canned fire-roasted diced tomatoes, drained

¼ cup tomato paste

2 tablespoons finely chopped fresh basil

½ teaspoon chopped garlic

Dash red pepper flakes

¼ teaspoon garlic powder

¼ teaspoon onion powder

¾ cup cubed eggplant

½ cup chopped red bell pepper

½ cup sliced and halved zucchini

⅓ cup roughly chopped onion

One 5-ounce fillet raw lean beefsteak

Dash each salt and black pepper

You'll Need: heavy-duty aluminum foil, baking sheet, nonstick spray, medium-large bowl, grill pan

Prep: 15 minutes

Cook: 30 minutes

1. Preheat oven to 375 degrees. Lay a large piece of heavy-duty foil on a baking sheet, and spray with nonstick spray.

2. In a medium-large bowl, combine tomatoes, tomato paste, basil, garlic, and red pepper flakes. Add ⅛ teaspoon each garlic powder and onion powder. Mix thoroughly.

3. Add all veggies to the bowl, and stir to coat. Distribute mixture onto the center of the foil.

4. Cover with another large piece of foil. Fold together and seal all four edges of the foil pieces, forming a well-sealed packet.

5. Bake for 25 minutes, or until veggies are tender.

6. About 15 minutes before veggies are done cooking, bring a grill pan sprayed with nonstick spray to medium-high heat. Season beef with salt, black pepper, and remaining ⅛ teaspoon each garlic powder and onion powder. Grill until cooked to your preference, 4 to 6 minutes per side.

7. Cut packet to release steam before opening entirely. Serve veggies with steak.

MAKES 1 SERVING

Apple Raisin Chicken Pack

Entire recipe: 330 calories, 7g fat, 424mg sodium, 31.5g carbs, 5g fiber, 20g sugars, 33g protein

1½ tablespoons balsamic vinegar

½ teaspoon brown sugar (not packed)

¾ teaspoon cornstarch

2 teaspoons light whipped butter or light buttery spread, room temperature

½ teaspoon Dijon mustard

4½ ounces raw boneless skinless chicken breast, cut into 1-inch cubes

Dash each salt and black pepper

½ cup chopped Fuji apple (or another sweet apple)

¼ cup chopped onion

1 tablespoon raisins, chopped

4 cups baby spinach leaves

You'll Need: heavy-duty aluminum foil, baking sheet, nonstick spray, 2 medium-large bowls, whisk

Prep: 15 minutes

Cook: 20 minutes

1. Preheat oven to 375 degrees. Lay a large piece of heavy-duty foil on a baking sheet, and spray with nonstick spray.

2. In a medium-large bowl, combine vinegar, sugar, and cornstarch. Whisk to dissolve. Add butter and mustard, and whisk until mostly uniform.

3. Season chicken with salt and pepper, and add to the bowl. Add apple, onion, and chopped raisins, and stir to coat.

4. Distribute mixture onto the center of foil. Cover with another large piece of foil.

5. Fold together and seal all four edges of the foil pieces, forming a well-sealed packet. Bake for 20 minutes, or until chicken is fully cooked and apple and onion are tender.

6. Meanwhile, place spinach in another medium-large bowl.

7. Cut packet to release steam before opening entirely. Add contents to the bowl of spinach, and mix well.

MAKES 1 SERVING

Chicken & Sweet Potato Pack

Entire recipe: 350 calories, 8.5g fat, 448mg sodium, 33g carbs, 5.5g fiber, 10g sugars, 35.5g protein

4 ounces sweet potato (about half of a medium potato), cut into 1-inch cubes

5 ounces raw boneless skinless chicken breast, cut into 1-inch cubes

1 cup zucchini cut into 1-inch chunks

⅓ cup chopped onion

1 teaspoon chopped garlic

2 dashes each salt and black pepper

1 teaspoon olive oil or grapeseed oil

You'll Need: heavy-duty aluminum foil, baking sheet, nonstick spray, medium-large microwave-safe bowl

Prep: 10 minutes

Cook: 25 minutes

1. Preheat oven to 375 degrees. Lay a large piece of heavy-duty foil on a baking sheet, and spray with nonstick spray.

2. Place cubed potato in a medium-large microwave-safe bowl. Add 1 tablespoon water, cover, and microwave for 2 minutes, or until slightly softened. Drain excess water.

3. Add remaining ingredients to the bowl, and mix well.

4. Distribute mixture onto the center of foil. Cover with another large piece of foil. Fold together and seal all four edges of the foil pieces, forming a well-sealed packet.

5. Bake for 20 minutes, or until chicken is cooked through and potatoes are tender. Cut packet to release steam before opening entirely.

MAKES 1 SERVING

Hawaiian Chicken Pack

Entire recipe: 347 calories, 9.5g fat, 706mg sodium, 28g carbs, 4g fiber, 18g sugars, 33.5g protein

5 ounces raw boneless skinless chicken breast, cut into 1-inch cubes

Dash each salt and black pepper

1 cup sliced red and yellow bell pepper

½ cup sliced onion

½ cup crushed pineapple packed in juice, lightly drained

2 tablespoons teriyaki sauce or marinade with 25 calories or less per tablespoon

1 teaspoon olive oil or grapeseed oil

You'll Need: heavy-duty aluminum foil, baking sheet, nonstick spray, large bowl

Prep: 10 minutes

Cook: 25 minutes

1. Preheat oven to 375 degrees. Lay a large piece of heavy-duty foil on a baking sheet, and spray with nonstick spray.

2. Place chicken in a large bowl, and season with salt and black pepper. Add remaining ingredients, and stir to coat.

3. Distribute mixture onto the center of the foil. Cover with another large piece of foil. Fold together and seal all four edges of the foil pieces, forming a well-sealed packet.

4. Bake for 25 minutes, or until chicken is cooked through and veggies have softened.

5. Cut packet to release steam before opening entirely.

MAKES 1 SERVING

Spicy BBQ Chicken Pack

Entire recipe: 350 calories, 9.5g fat, 652mg sodium, 30g carbs, 7g fiber, 13g sugars, 39.5g protein

2 tablespoons BBQ sauce with 45 calories or less per 2-tablespoon serving

1 teaspoon Sriracha sauce

1 teaspoon olive oil or grapeseed oil

1 teaspoon chopped garlic

Dash garlic powder

Dash onion powder

Dash black pepper

3 cups small broccoli florets

5 ounces raw boneless skinless chicken breast, cut into 1-inch cubes

You'll Need: heavy-duty aluminum foil, baking sheet, nonstick spray, large bowl

Prep: 10 minutes

Cook: 20 minutes

1. Preheat oven to 375 degrees. Lay a large piece of heavy-duty foil on a baking sheet, and spray with nonstick spray.

2. In a large bowl, combine all ingredients *except* broccoli and chicken. Mix until uniform. Add broccoli and chicken, and stir to coat.

3. Distribute mixture onto the center of the foil. Cover with another large piece of foil. Fold together and seal all four edges of the foil pieces, forming a well-sealed packet.

4. Bake for 20 minutes, or until chicken is cooked through and broccoli has softened.

5. Cut packet to release steam before opening entirely.

MAKES 1 SERVING

HG-ified Fish 'n Chips

Entire recipe: 340 calories, 8g fat, 646mg sodium, 40g carbs, 12g fiber, 12.5g sugars, 34g protein

CHIPS

6 ounces peeled carrots (about 1 large carrot), cut into French-fry-shaped spears

1 teaspoon olive oil or grapeseed oil

Dash salt

1 tablespoon ketchup

(continued on next page)

You'll Need: baking sheet, nonstick spray, medium bowl, 2 wide bowls

Prep: 15 minutes

Cook: 20 minutes

1. Preheat oven to 425 degrees. Spray a baking sheet with nonstick spray.

2. In a medium bowl, drizzle carrot spears with oil, and toss to coat.

3. Lay spears on the baking sheet, and bake for 10 minutes.

FISH

¼ cup Fiber One Original bran cereal, finely crushed

2 tablespoons panko breadcrumbs

¼ teaspoon salt-free seasoning mix

¼ teaspoon garlic powder

⅛ teaspoon onion powder

⅛ teaspoon black pepper

¼ cup egg whites or fat-free liquid egg substitute

One 5-ounce raw tilapia, cod, or sea bass fillet

4. Meanwhile, in a wide bowl, combine cereal crumbs, breadcrumbs, and all seasonings. Mix well. Place egg whites/substitute in another wide bowl.

5. Remove sheet from oven, and flip carrot spears, arranging them on one half of the sheet (leaving room for the fish).

6. Gently dunk fish into the egg, shake to remove excess, and coat with crumb mixture. Lay fish alongside carrot spears on the baking sheet.

7. Bake until carrot spears and fish are cooked through and slightly crispy, about 10 more minutes.

8. Sprinkle carrot spears with salt, and serve with ketchup for dipping.

MAKES 1 SERVING

HG Alternative

If you can't find a 5-ounce fish fillet, use two smaller fillets that total 5 ounces.

Foil Packs & HG Bakes   **221**

Southwest Chicken Bake
with buttered corn 📷

Entire recipe: 337 calories, 9.5g fat, 670mg sodium, 30.5g carbs, 3.5g fiber, 8g sugars, 33g protein

¼ cup sliced onion

¼ cup sliced green bell pepper

2 teaspoons taco seasoning mix

One 4-ounce raw boneless skinless chicken breast cutlet, pounded to ¼-inch thickness

1½ tablespoons shredded reduced-fat Mexican-blend cheese

One frozen 7-inch ear of sweet yellow corn *or* ⅔ cup frozen sweet corn kernels

1¼ teaspoons light whipped butter or light buttery spread

2 tablespoons salsa/ pico de gallo with 90mg sodium or less per 2-tablespoon serving

1 tablespoon light sour cream

You'll Need: 8-inch by 8-inch baking pan, nonstick spray, skillet, aluminum foil

Prep: 15 minutes

Cook: 35 minutes

1. Preheat oven to 350 degrees. Spray an 8-inch by 8-inch baking pan with nonstick spray.

2. Bring a skillet sprayed with nonstick spray to medium-high heat. Add onion, pepper, 1 teaspoon taco seasoning, and 2 tablespoons water. Cook and stir until water has evaporated and veggies have softened, about 3 minutes.

3. Season chicken cutlet with remaining 1 teaspoon taco seasoning. Place cooked veggies in the center of the chicken cutlet, and roll up the cutlet over the veggies. If needed, secure with toothpicks.

4. Place stuffed chicken in the pan. Cover pan with foil, and bake for 15 minutes.

5. Remove foil, and sprinkle chicken with cheese. Bake until chicken is cooked through, about 15 minutes.

6. Meanwhile, heat corn in the microwave according to package instructions. Spread or mix with butter.

7. Top chicken with salsa/pico de gallo and sour cream, and serve with buttered corn.

MAKES 1 SERVING

For the latest food news, recipes, tips 'n tricks, and more, **sign up for free daily emails at hungry-girl.com!**

Italian Chicken Bake
with veggies marinara

Entire recipe: 350 calories, 10g fat, 457mg sodium, 27.5g carbs, 8.5g fiber, 13g sugars, 37g protein

⅓ cup thinly sliced onion

⅓ cup thinly sliced green bell pepper

1 teaspoon olive oil or grapeseed oil

2½ tablespoons low-fat/light ricotta cheese

¾ teaspoon salt-free seasoning mix

¼ teaspoon onion powder

¼ teaspoon garlic powder

One 4-ounce raw boneless skinless chicken breast cutlet, pounded to ¼-inch thickness

1 cup broccoli florets

1 cup cauliflower florets

½ cup canned crushed tomatoes

⅛ teaspoon Italian seasoning

1 teaspoon grated Parmesan cheese

You'll Need: 8-inch by 8-inch baking pan, nonstick spray, skillet, 2 medium bowls, aluminum foil

Prep: 10 minutes

Cook: 40 minutes

1. Preheat oven to 350 degrees. Spray an 8-inch by 8-inch baking pan with nonstick spray.

2. Bring a skillet sprayed with nonstick spray to medium-high heat. Add onion and bell pepper, and drizzle with oil. Cook and stir until slightly softened and lightly browned, about 3 minutes.

3. Transfer onion and pepper to a medium bowl. Add ricotta cheese, ¼ teaspoon salt-free seasoning, and ⅛ teaspoon each onion powder and garlic powder. Mix thoroughly.

4. Season chicken cutlet with remaining ½ teaspoon salt-free seasoning. Place veggie-cheese mixture in the center of the chicken cutlet, and roll up the cutlet over the mixture. If needed, secure with toothpicks.

5. Place stuffed chicken in the pan, and place broccoli and cauliflower alongside it. Cover pan with foil, and bake for 20 minutes.

6. Meanwhile, in another medium bowl, combine crushed tomatoes, Italian seasoning, and remaining ⅛ teaspoon each onion powder and garlic powder. Mix well.

7. Remove foil, and bake until chicken is cooked through and veggies have softened, about 15 minutes.

8. Spoon 2 tablespoons of the seasoned tomatoes over the chicken. Toss veggies in the remaining tomatoes, and sprinkle with Parm.

MAKES 1 SERVING

Meatloaf 'n Mashies 📷

¼ of recipe (2 slices meatloaf with about 1 cup mashies): 334 calories, 8.5 fat, 750mg sodium, 28.5g carbs, 9g fiber, 11.5g sugars, 36.5g protein

MEATLOAF

1½ cups chopped portabella mushrooms

1 pound raw extra-lean ground beef (4% fat or less)

½ cup canned crushed tomatoes

½ cup old-fashioned oats

¼ cup egg whites or fat-free liquid egg substitute

½ teaspoon onion powder

½ teaspoon garlic powder

¼ teaspoon each salt and black pepper

2 tablespoons ketchup

(continued on next page)

You'll Need: 9-inch by 5-inch loaf pan, nonstick spray, skillet, large bowl, large microwave-safe bowl

Prep: 25 minutes

Cook: 1 hour

1. Preheat oven to 400 degrees. Spray a 9-inch by 5-inch loaf pan with nonstick spray.

2. Bring a skillet sprayed with nonstick spray to medium-high heat. Cook and stir mushrooms until completely softened, about 5 minutes.

3. Transfer mushrooms to a large bowl, and blot away excess moisture. Add all remaining meatloaf ingredients *except* ketchup. Mix thoroughly.

4. Transfer mixture to the loaf pan, and smooth out the surface. Evenly top with ketchup.

5. Bake until cooked through, about 50 minutes.

MASHIES

10 cups frozen cauliflower florets

3 wedges The Laughing Cow Light Creamy Swiss cheese

½ teaspoon garlic powder

½ teaspoon onion powder

⅛ teaspoon each salt and black pepper

2 tablespoons grated Parmesan cheese

6. About 20 minutes before meatloaf is done, place cauliflower in a large microwave-safe bowl. Add ¼ cup water, cover, and microwave for 8 minutes. Uncover and stir. Re-cover and microwave for 8 minutes, or until soft.

7. Drain excess liquid from cauliflower. Add cheese wedges, breaking them into pieces. Add all remaining mashie ingredients *except* Parm. Thoroughly mash and mix. Stir in Parm.

8. Cut meatloaf into eight slices, and serve with mashies.

MAKES 4 SERVINGS

HG Tip!

For extra-creamy mashies, blend them in a blender or food processor until smooth.

Eggplant 'Bella Chicken Tower

Entire recipe: 330 calories, 8.5g fat, 660mg sodium, 29g carbs, 9g fiber, 14g sugars, 36.5g protein

Three ½-inch-thick eggplant slices (cut widthwise from the center of a medium eggplant)

Two portabella mushroom caps (stems removed)

One 4.5-ounce raw boneless skinless chicken breast cutlet, pounded to ½-inch thickness

¼ teaspoon garlic powder

¼ teaspoon onion powder

¼ teaspoon each salt and black pepper

2½ tablespoons balsamic vinegar

1 teaspoon olive oil or grapeseed oil

You'll Need: baking sheet, nonstick spray, plate, small bowl, whisk

Prep: 10 minutes

Cook: 25 minutes

1. Preheat oven to 350 degrees. Spray a baking sheet with nonstick spray.

2. Sprinkle eggplant, mushroom caps, and chicken with seasonings. Place on the baking sheet, with the rounded sides of the mushroom caps down.

3. Bake for 10 minutes.

4. Flip contents of the sheet. Bake until veggies have softened and chicken is cooked through, about 15 minutes.

5. Stack ingredients on a plate in the following order: eggplant slice, mushroom cap, eggplant slice, chicken breast, mushroom cap, eggplant slice.

6. In a small bowl, whisk vinegar with oil. Drizzle over stack.

MAKES 1 SERVING

Southwest Super-Stuffed Pepper

Entire recipe: 333 calories, 9.5g fat, 605mg sodium, 35.5g carbs, 8g fiber, 13.5g sugars, 29g protein

1 large green bell pepper (look for one that sits flat when stem end is up)

3 ounces raw lean ground turkey (7% fat or less)

¼ teaspoon garlic powder

⅛ teaspoon chili powder

Dash each salt and black pepper

1 cup chopped brown mushrooms

1 cup chopped broccoli

¼ cup chopped onion

3 tablespoons frozen sweet corn kernels

2 tablespoons canned black beans, drained and rinsed

2 tablespoons shredded reduced-fat Mexican-blend cheese

¼ cup salsa with 90mg sodium or less per 2-tablespoon serving

You'll Need: loaf pan, large skillet, nonstick spray

Prep: 10 minutes

Cook: 35 minutes

1. Preheat oven to 350 degrees.

2. Carefully slice off and discard the stem end of the bell pepper (about ½ inch). Remove and discard seeds.

3. Place pepper cut side up in a loaf pan. If pepper does not sit flat, gently lean it against side of the pan for support.

4. Bake until tender, 30 to 35 minutes.

5. Meanwhile, bring a large skillet sprayed with nonstick spray to medium-high heat. Add turkey, and sprinkle with seasonings. Add mushrooms, broccoli, onion, corn, and beans. Cook, stir, and crumble until turkey is fully cooked and veggies have softened, 5 to 7 minutes. Remove from heat, and stir in cheese and salsa. Cover to keep warm.

6. Blot away excess moisture from bell pepper. Fill pepper with turkey mixture.

MAKES 1 SERVING

Chicken Veggie Pizza
with side salad 📷

Entire recipe: 348 calories, 8g fat, 722mg sodium, 40g carbs, 10g fiber, 9.5g sugars, 36.5g protein

PIZZA

1 medium-large high-fiber flour tortilla with 110 calories or less

3 tablespoons canned crushed tomatoes

⅛ teaspoon garlic powder, or more to taste

⅛ teaspoon onion powder, or more to taste

Dash Italian seasoning

3 tablespoons shredded part-skim mozzarella cheese

3 ounces cooked and chopped skinless chicken breast

2 tablespoons finely chopped bell pepper

2 tablespoons finely chopped mushrooms

2 tablespoons finely chopped onion

You'll Need: baking sheet, nonstick spray, small bowl, medium bowl

Prep: 10 minutes

Cook: 10 minutes

1. Preheat oven to 375 degrees. Spray a baking sheet with nonstick spray.

2. Lay tortilla on the sheet, and bake until slightly crispy, about 5 minutes.

3. Meanwhile, in a small bowl, stir seasonings into crushed tomatoes.

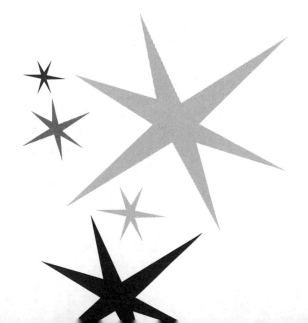

SIDE SALAD

1 cup lettuce

1 cup cucumber, mushrooms, and/or other high-volume veggies (page 345)

1 tablespoon salsa or pico de gallo with 90mg sodium or less per 2-tablespoon serving

2 teaspoons vinegar (balsamic, red wine, white wine, rice, or cider)

4. Flip tortilla. Spread with seasoned tomatoes, leaving a ½-inch border. Top with cheese, chicken, and veggies.

5. Bake until cheese has melted, toppings are hot, and tortilla is crisp, about 5 more minutes.

6. Toss salad ingredients in a medium bowl, and serve with pizza.

MAKES 1 SERVING

Shrimp 'n Veggie White Pizza

Entire recipe: 330 calories, 8g fat, 729mg sodium, 38.5g carbs, 8.5g fiber, 10.5g sugars, 32g protein

1 medium-large high-fiber flour tortilla with 110 calories or less

⅓ cup light/low-fat ricotta cheese

1 tablespoon shredded part-skim mozzarella cheese

¼ teaspoon garlic powder

Dash black pepper

4 slices plum tomato

4 fresh basil leaves

½ cup sliced red bell pepper

⅓ cup sliced onion

3 ounces (about 6) raw large shrimp, peeled, tails removed, deveined, chopped into bite-sized pieces

You'll Need: baking sheet, nonstick spray, small bowl, skillet

Prep: 10 minutes

Cook: 15 minutes

1. Preheat oven to 375 degrees. Spray a baking sheet with nonstick spray.

2. Lay tortilla on the baking sheet, and bake until slightly crispy, about 5 minutes.

3. Meanwhile, in a small bowl, combine ricotta cheese, mozzarella cheese, garlic powder, and black pepper. Mix well.

4. Flip tortilla. Spread with cheese mixture, leaving a ½-inch border. Top with tomato and basil.

5. Bake until crispy, 3 to 4 minutes.

6. Bring a skillet sprayed with nonstick spray to medium-high heat. Add bell pepper and onion. Cook and stir until partially softened, about 3 minutes.

7. Add shrimp to the skillet. Cook and stir until shrimp are cooked through and veggies have softened, about 3 minutes.

8. Evenly top pizza with shrimp and veggies.

MAKES 1 SERVING

Turkey-Stuffed Portabella
with BBQ slaw

Entire recipe: 342 calories, 8g fat, 523mg sodium, 38g carbs, 11g fiber, 19.5g sugars, 33.5g protein

2½ cups bagged broccoli cole slaw

1 portabella mushroom, stem chopped and reserved

4 ounces raw lean ground turkey (7% fat or less)

¼ teaspoon garlic powder

Dash black pepper

⅓ cup diced onion

2 tablespoons BBQ sauce with 45 calories or less per 2-tablespoon serving

¼ cup diced tomato

1 tablespoon fat-free plain Greek yogurt

You'll Need: baking sheet, nonstick spray, medium microwave-safe bowl, skillet

Prep: 10 minutes

Cook: 20 minutes

1. Preheat oven to 400 degrees. Spray a baking sheet with nonstick spray.

2. Place broccoli slaw in a medium microwave-safe bowl. Add 2 tablespoons water, cover, and microwave for 3 minutes, or until softened. Drain excess water, and cover to keep warm.

3. Place mushroom cap on the sheet, rounded side down. Bake until tender, about 15 minutes.

4. Meanwhile, bring a skillet sprayed with nonstick spray to medium-high heat. Add turkey, and sprinkle with garlic powder and pepper. Add onion and chopped mushroom stem. Cook, stir, and crumble until turkey is fully cooked and veggies have softened, 5 to 7 minutes. Remove from heat, and stir in 1 tablespoon BBQ sauce.

5. Blot away excess moisture from mushroom cap. Fill with turkey mixture. Top with tomato and Greek yogurt.

6. Stir remaining 1 tablespoon BBQ sauce into the slaw. Serve with stuffed mushroom.

MAKES 1 SERVING

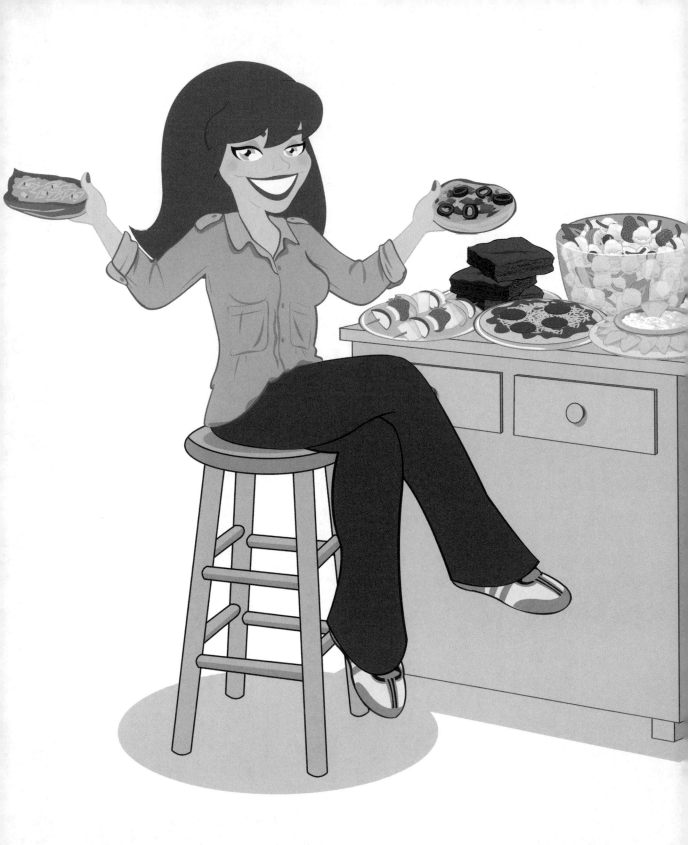

Snacks

Crispy, Crunchy

Everyone craves some CRUNCH now
and then. From flavor-packed cracker
stacks to MUST-TRY veggie chips,
these snacks are AWESOME!

Easy Caprese Crisps

Entire recipe: 97 calories, 3.5g fat, 230mg sodium, 11.5g carbs, 1.5g fiber, 2g sugars, 5g protein

4 Old London Roasted Garlic Melba Snacks

2 slices plum tomato, halved

1 tablespoon chopped fresh basil

1½ tablespoons shredded part-skim mozzarella cheese

You'll Need: microwave-safe plate

Prep: 5 minutes

Cook: 5 minutes or less

1. On a microwave-safe plate, top each Melba Snack with half a slice of tomato. Top with basil, and sprinkle with cheese.

2. Microwave for 30 seconds, or until cheese has just melted.

MAKES 1 SERVING

Deli-Style Turkey Toasts

Entire recipe: 98 calories, 0.5g fat, 250mg sodium, 13.5g carbs, 0g fiber, 0g sugars, 9.5g protein

1 ounce (1 to 2 slices) no-salt-added turkey

3 Old London Classic Melba Toasts

1 teaspoon Dijon mustard

Prep: 5 minutes

Tear turkey into pieces, and distribute among Toasts. Evenly top with mustard.

MAKES 1 SERVING

Cheese 'n Tomato Toasts

Entire recipe: 100 calories, 1.5g fat, 181mg sodium, 15.5g carbs, 2g fiber, 1.5g sugars, 5g protein

3 Old London Salt Free Whole Grain Melba Toasts

1 wedge The Laughing Cow Light Creamy Swiss cheese

⅛ teaspoon Italian seasoning

⅛ teaspoon garlic powder

1 large tomato slice, cut into 3 wedges

Prep: 5 minutes

Spread Toasts with cheese, and sprinkle with Italian seasoning and garlic powder. Top each with a piece of tomato.

MAKES 1 SERVING

Zesty Tuna Crunchcake

Entire recipe: 99 calories, 0.5g fat, 95mg sodium, 10.5g carbs, 0.5g fiber, 2g sugars, 12.5g protein

1½ ounces low-sodium tuna packed in water (drained)

2 tablespoons finely chopped bell pepper

1 tablespoon finely chopped onion

1 tablespoon salsa with 90mg sodium or less per 2-tablespoon serving

Dash chili powder

Dash garlic powder

1 lightly salted rice cake

You'll Need: medium bowl

Prep: 5 minutes

1. In a medium bowl, combine all ingredients *except* the rice cake. Mix well.

2. Spoon mixture over the rice cake.

MAKES 1 SERVING

View B4 You Chew: Veggie Chip Tips!

Cutting your veggies with a mandoline slicer is a must. The handy kitchen tool can thinly slice perfectly uniform pieces. And these chips are so good, it's worth picking one up!

During the last 30 minutes of cook time, check on chips often, and remove those that are done.

To get them as crispy as possible, cool them on a cooling rack!

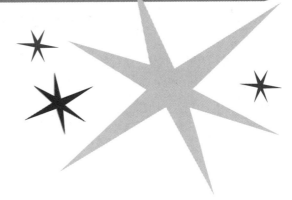

Zucchini Chips 📷

Entire recipe: 95 calories, 3.5g fat, 191mg sodium, 16g carbs, 4.5g fiber, 11.5g sugars, 5.5g protein

1 pound (about 2 medium) zucchini

Dash salt

You'll Need: 2 baking sheets, olive oil nonstick spray, mandoline slicer

Prep: 5 minutes

Cook: 1 hour and 45 minutes

1. Preheat oven to 250 degrees. Spray two baking sheets with olive oil nonstick spray.

2. Using a mandoline slicer, cut zucchini into ⅛-inch-thick rounds.

3. Lay zucchini rounds on the sheets, evenly spaced. Cover with a 2-second spray of the olive oil spray, and sprinkle with salt.

4. Bake for 45 minutes.

5. Carefully remove baking sheets, and return them to the oven on the opposite racks.

6. Bake until zucchini rounds are golden brown and dry to the touch, about 1 hour.

7. Let cool completely.

MAKES 1 SERVING

Parsnip Chips 📷

Entire recipe: 100 calories, 2g fat, 166mg sodium, 20.5g carbs, 5.5g fiber, 5.5g sugars, 1.5g protein

4 ounces parsnip (about ¼ of a large parsnip)

Dash salt

You'll Need: baking sheet, olive oil nonstick spray, mandoline slicer

Prep: 5 minutes

Cook: 1 hour and 30 minutes

1. Preheat oven to 250 degrees. Spray a baking sheet with olive oil nonstick spray.

2. Using a mandoline slicer, cut parsnip into rounds, about ⅛ inch thick.

3. Lay parsnip rounds on the sheet, evenly spaced. Cover with a 2-second spray of the olive oil spray, and sprinkle with salt.

4. Bake until parsnip rounds are golden brown, dry, and firm to the touch, about 1½ hours.

5. Let cool completely.

MAKES 1 SERVING

Parsnip Tips!

Choose a parsnip that's more round than narrow. Bigger chips = better. And treat this root veggie like you would a potato: Scrub it clean! Same goes for beets . . .

Beet Chips 📷

Entire recipe: 100 calories, 2g fat, 155mg sodium, 19g carbs, 5.5g fiber, 13.5g sugars, 3g protein

7 ounces (1 to 2) beets

You'll Need: baking sheet, olive oil nonstick spray, mandoline slicer

Prep: 5 minutes

Cook: 1 hour and 30 minutes

1. Preheat oven to 250 degrees. Spray a baking sheet with olive oil nonstick spray.

2. Using a mandoline slicer, cut beets into ⅛-inch-thick rounds.

3. Lay beet rounds on the sheet, evenly spaced. Cover with a 2-second spray of the olive oil spray.

4. Bake until beet rounds are shriveled and dry to the touch, about 1½ hours.

5. Let cool completely.

MAKES 1 SERVING

Faux-Fried Zucchini

Entire recipe: 100 calories, 3g fat, 183mg sodium, 20g carbs, 7.5g fiber, 7g sugars, 7.5g protein

3 tablespoons Fiber One Original cereal, finely crushed

½ teaspoon garlic powder

½ teaspoon onion powder

Dash black pepper

2 cups zucchini sliced into ½-inch-thick rounds

1 tablespoon egg whites or fat-free liquid egg substitute

2 teaspoons grated Parmesan cheese

You'll Need: baking sheet, nonstick spray, wide bowl, medium bowl

Prep: 15 minutes

Cook: 20 minutes

1. Preheat oven to 375 degrees. Spray a baking sheet with nonstick spray.

2. In a wide bowl, combine crushed cereal with seasonings. Mix well.

3. Place zucchini rounds in a medium bowl, top with egg white/substitute, and toss to coat. One at a time, shake zucchini rounds to remove excess egg, thoroughly coat with crumbs, and place on the baking sheet.

4. Evenly top zucchini rounds with Parm.

5. Bake until outsides are lightly browned and insides are soft, about 20 minutes.

MAKES 1 SERVING

Bell Pepper Strips with Black Bean Dip

Entire recipe: 97 calories, 0.5g fat, 218mg sodium, 16.5g carbs, 5g fiber, 5g sugars, 7g protein

¼ cup canned black beans, drained and rinsed

2 tablespoons fat-free plain Greek yogurt

1 tablespoon canned green chiles

Dash onion powder

Dash garlic powder

Dash ground cumin

Dash chili powder

1 cup bell pepper cut into 1-inch-wide slices

You'll Need: small bowl

Prep: 10 minutes

1. In a small bowl, combine beans, yogurt, and green chiles. Mash until chunky but well mixed. Stir in seasonings.

2. Serve with pepper slices for dipping.

MAKES 1 SERVING

Pizza, Pizza

One can NEVER have too many
ways to satisfy a pizza craving.
And for a mealtime fix, don't miss
the Chicken Veggie Pizza on
page 230 and the Shrimp 'n Veggie
White Pizza on page 232!

Pepperoni Pizza-bella

Entire recipe: 93 calories, 3.5g fat, 238mg sodium, 9g carbs, 2.5g fiber, 3.5g sugars, 8.5g protein

1 portabella mushroom, stem chopped and reserved

2 tablespoons canned crushed tomatoes

⅛ teaspoon garlic powder

Dash onion powder

Dash Italian seasoning

2 tablespoons shredded part-skim mozzarella cheese

2 slices turkey pepperoni, chopped

Optional topping: red pepper flakes

You'll Need: baking sheet, nonstick spray, small bowl

Prep: 5 minutes

Cook: 20 minutes

1. Preheat oven to 400 degrees. Spray a baking sheet with nonstick spray.

2. Place mushroom cap on the sheet, rounded side down. Bake until slightly tender, about 8 minutes.

3. Meanwhile, in a small bowl, stir seasonings into crushed tomatoes. Add chopped mushroom stem, and mix well.

4. Remove sheet, but leave oven on.

5. Blot away excess moisture from mushroom cap. Evenly top with tomato mixture. Sprinkle with cheese and chopped pepperoni.

6. Bake until mushroom is tender, tomato mixture is hot, and cheese has melted, 8 to 10 minutes.

MAKES 1 SERVING

Mini Pizza-Stuffed Mushrooms

Entire recipe: 96 calories, 3g fat, 229mg sodium, 9.5g carbs, 2g fiber, 4.5g sugars, 9.5g protein

6 medium baby bella mushroom caps (each about 2 inches wide), stems removed

2 tablespoons chopped bell pepper

1 tablespoon chopped onion

2 tablespoons canned crushed tomatoes

⅛ teaspoon garlic powder

Dash onion powder

Dash Italian seasoning

1 piece Mini Babybel Light cheese, finely chopped

Optional topping: red pepper flakes

You'll Need: baking sheet, nonstick spray, microwave-safe mug (or small microwave-safe bowl)

Prep: 5 minutes

Cook: 15 minutes

1. Preheat oven to 375 degrees. Spray a baking sheet with nonstick spray.

2. Place mushroom caps on the sheet, rounded sides down. Bake until tender, 8 to 10 minutes. Remove sheet, but leave oven on.

3. Meanwhile, place pepper and onion in a microwave-safe mug (or small microwave-safe bowl) sprayed with nonstick spray. Microwave for 1 minute, or until softened. Add crushed tomatoes and seasonings, and mix well.

4. Blot away excess moisture from mushroom caps. Evenly distribute tomato mixture among the mushroom caps, and sprinkle with chopped cheese.

5. Bake until filling is hot and cheese has melted, about 3 minutes.

MAKES 1 SERVING

Quickie Tortilla Pizza

Entire recipe: 100 calories, 3.5g fat, 145mg sodium, 12.5g carbs, 1.5g fiber, 1.5g sugars, 5g protein

One 6-inch corn tortilla

1½ tablespoons canned crushed tomatoes

Dash garlic powder, or more to taste

Dash onion powder, or more to taste

Dash Italian seasoning, or more to taste

2 tablespoons shredded part-skim mozzarella cheese

Optional topping: red pepper flakes

You'll Need: baking sheet, nonstick spray, small bowl

Prep: 5 minutes

Cook: 15 minutes

1. Preheat oven to 375 degrees. Spray a baking sheet with nonstick spray.

2. Lay tortilla on the baking sheet, and bake until slightly crispy, about 5 minutes.

3. Meanwhile, in a small bowl, stir seasonings into crushed tomatoes.

4. Flip tortilla, and spread with seasoned tomatoes, leaving a ½-inch border. Sprinkle with cheese.

5. Bake until hot and lightly browned, 5 to 7 minutes.

MAKES 1 SERVING

Easy English-Muffin Pizza

Entire recipe: 99 calories, 3g fat, 225mg sodium, 14.5g carbs, 3.5g fiber, 1.5g sugars, 6.5g protein

1½ tablespoons canned crushed tomatoes

Dash Italian seasoning

Dash onion powder

Dash garlic powder

Half of a light English muffin

2 tablespoons shredded part-skim mozzarella cheese

Optional topping: red pepper flakes

You'll Need: baking sheet, nonstick spray, small bowl

Prep: 5 minutes

Cook: 5 minutes

1. Preheat oven to 400 degrees. Spray a baking sheet with nonstick spray.

2. In a small bowl, stir seasonings into crushed tomatoes. Spread seasoned tomatoes onto the English muffin half, and sprinkle with cheese. Transfer to the baking sheet.

3. Bake until English muffin is crisp on the edges and cheese has melted, about 5 minutes.

MAKES 1 SERVING

HG Alternative

Whip this up in a toaster oven!

Soups, Salads & Slaws

These veggie-packed snacks are large and in charge! Spoon or spear your way to satisfaction . . .

Giant Noodle Soup Bowl

¼ of recipe (about 2 cups): 85 calories, 1g fat, 217mg sodium, 16g carbs, 4g fiber, 6g sugars, 5g protein

1 bag House Foods Tofu Shirataki Spaghetti Shaped Noodle Substitute

2 cups sliced mushrooms

1 cup chopped onion

1 cup chopped carrots

1 tablespoon chopped garlic

6 cups low-sodium chicken or vegetable broth

1 cup chopped celery

½ cup frozen peas

¼ teaspoon ground ginger

¼ teaspoon red pepper flakes

Optional seasoning: salt-free seasoning mix

You'll Need: strainer, large microwave-safe bowl, large pot with a lid, nonstick spray

Prep: 10 minutes

Cook: 30 minutes

1. Use a strainer to rinse and drain noodles. Thoroughly pat dry. Roughly cut noodles, and transfer to a large microwave-safe bowl. Microwave for 2 minutes. Drain excess liquid, and thoroughly pat dry.

2. Bring a large pot sprayed with nonstick spray to medium heat. Add mushrooms, onion, carrots, and garlic. Cook and stir until veggies have slightly softened, about 5 minutes.

3. Carefully add noodles and remaining ingredients. Mix well, and bring to a boil.

4. Reduce to a simmer. Cover and cook for 15 minutes, or until veggies have softened.

MAKES 4 SERVINGS

Pumpkin Veggie Soup 📷

¼ of recipe (about 2 cups): 100 calories, 0.5g fat, 218mg sodium, 18.5g carbs, 6.5g fiber, 6.5g sugars, 6.5g protein

2 cups chopped zucchini

1½ cups chopped celery

⅔ cup chopped bell pepper

1 teaspoon salt-free seasoning mix

5 cups low-sodium chicken or vegetable broth

1 cup canned pure pumpkin

¼ teaspoon garlic powder

¼ teaspoon onion powder

⅛ teaspoon paprika

⅛ teaspoon chili powder

⅔ cup canned white kidney beans (cannellini beans), drained and rinsed

You'll Need: large pot with a lid, nonstick spray

Prep: 10 minutes

Cook: 30 minutes

1. Bring a large pot sprayed with nonstick spray to medium-high heat. Add zucchini, celery, bell pepper, and salt-free seasoning. Cook and stir until veggies have softened and browned, about 8 minutes.

2. Carefully add all remaining ingredients *except* beans. Mix well, and bring to a boil.

3. Reduce to a simmer. Cover and cook for 15 minutes.

4. Stir in beans, and cook until hot, about 1 minute.

MAKES 4 SERVINGS

📷 Photo Alert!

The camera icon next to the recipe name means flip to the insert to see a photo of this recipe. Find full-color photos of ALL the recipes at hungry-girl.com/books.

Perfect Pureed Veggie Soup

⅕ of recipe (about 1¾ cups): 93 calories, 0.5g fat, 173mg sodium, 18g carbs, 6g fiber, 6.5g sugars, 5.5g protein

2 cups chopped carrots

1 cup chopped onion

1½ teaspoons salt-free seasoning mix

4 cups chopped broccoli

4 cups chopped cauliflower

3 cups low-sodium vegetable broth

1 tablespoon chopped garlic

⅛ teaspoon each salt and black pepper

You'll Need: large pot with a lid, nonstick spray, blender

Prep: 20 minutes

Cook: 35 minutes

Cool: 10 minutes

1. Bring a large pot sprayed with nonstick spray to medium-high heat. Add carrots, onion, and salt-free seasoning. Cook and stir until softened and browned, about 8 minutes.

2. Add remaining veggies, broth, garlic, and 3 cups water. Mix well, and bring to a boil.

3. Reduce to a simmer. Cover and cook for 15 minutes.

4. Remove from heat, and let cool for 10 minutes.

5. Working in batches, carefully transfer contents of the pot to a blender, and puree until smooth. Stir in salt and pepper.

MAKES 5 SERVINGS

HG Tip!

Love big-batch pureed soups like this one? A handheld immersion blender is a great little investment—you can puree the soup right in the pot.

Super Sunomono Salad

Entire recipe: 95 calories, 0.5g fat, 164mg sodium, 23.5g carbs, 2g fiber, 15.5g sugars, 2.5g protein

3 tablespoons plain rice vinegar (not seasoned)

2 teaspoons granulated sugar

Dash salt

4 cups thinly sliced cucumber

You'll Need: small bowl, large bowl or sealable bag

Prep: 5 minutes

Chill: 1 hour or more (optional)

1. In a small bowl, combine vinegar, sugar, and salt. Stir until sugar and salt have dissolved.

2. Place cucumber in a large bowl (if eating immediately) or sealable bag (if marinating). Add vinegar mixture, and either stir to coat or seal the bag, removing as much air as possible.

3. If you like, marinate in the fridge for 1 hour or more. (The longer it marinates, the better it tastes.)

MAKES 1 SERVING

Southwest Snack Slaw

¼ of recipe (about 1¼ cups): 92 calories, 0.5g fat, 165mg sodium, 11.5g carbs, 4g fiber, 4.5g sugars, 11g protein

½ cup salsa or pico de gallo with 90mg sodium or less per 2-tablespoon serving

¼ cup fat-free plain Greek yogurt

2 tablespoons chopped cilantro

¼ teaspoon ground cumin

¼ teaspoon garlic powder

One 12-ounce bag (4 cups) broccoli cole slaw

4 ounces cooked and chopped skinless chicken breast

½ cup chopped jicama

¼ cup frozen sweet corn kernels, thawed

You'll Need: large bowl

Prep: 10 minutes

---

1. In a large bowl, combine salsa/pico de gallo, yogurt, cilantro, cumin, and garlic powder. Stir until uniform.

2. Add remaining ingredients, and stir to coat.

MAKES 4 SERVINGS

More Savory Snacks

What do these recipes have in common? They're easy, delicious, and SO satisfying!

Cheesy Bell Pepper Bites

Entire recipe: 99 calories, 4g fat, 228mg sodium, 12g carbs, 3g fiber, 6.5g sugars, 6g protein

1 bell pepper, quartered lengthwise, stem and seeds removed

⅛ teaspoon chili powder

⅛ teaspoon ground cumin

⅛ teaspoon paprika

2½ tablespoons shredded reduced-fat Mexican-blend cheese

2 tablespoons salsa or pico de gallo with 90mg sodium or less per 2-tablespoon serving

You'll Need: baking sheet, nonstick spray

Prep: 5 minutes

Cook: 15 minutes

1. Preheat oven to 375 degrees. Spray a baking sheet with nonstick spray.

2. Place bell pepper pieces on the sheet, cut sides up. Sprinkle with seasonings.

3. Bake until softened slightly, about 10 minutes.

4. Top with cheese, and bake until melted, about 1 minute.

5. Top with salsa/pico de gallo.

MAKES 1 SERVING

Creamy Avocado Fettuccine

Entire recipe: 100 calories, 6.5g fat, 212mg sodium, 9.5g carbs, 6g fiber, 1g sugars, 3g protein

1 bag House Foods Shirataki Fettuccine Shaped Noodle Substitute

1 wedge The Laughing Cow Light Creamy Swiss cheese

1 ounce (about 2 tablespoons) mashed avocado

⅛ teaspoon garlic powder, or more to taste

Dash dried basil, or more to taste

Dash black pepper, or more to taste

You'll Need: strainer, microwave-safe bowl

Prep: 5 minutes

Cook: 5 minutes or less

1. Use a strainer to rinse and drain noodles. Thoroughly pat dry. Roughly cut noodles, and transfer to a microwave-safe bowl. Microwave for 1 minute. Thoroughly pat dry.

2. Add remaining ingredients, breaking the cheese wedge into pieces, and stir until well mixed. Microwave for 1 minute. Stir well.

MAKES 1 SERVING

For the latest food news, recipes, tips 'n tricks, and more, **sign up for free daily emails at hungry-girl.com!**

Mexi-Tuna Lettuce Cups

Entire recipe: 100 calories, 1g fat, 78mg sodium, 5g carbs, 1g fiber, 2.5g sugars, 18g protein

One 2.6-ounce pouch low-sodium tuna packed in water

⅛ teaspoon ground cumin

⅛ teaspoon chili powder

⅛ teaspoon garlic powder

¼ cup chopped tomato

2 tablespoons finely chopped red onion

1 tablespoon finely chopped cilantro

2 medium butter lettuce leaves (or other round lettuce leaves)

Optional seasoning: salt-free seasoning mix

You'll Need: medium bowl

Prep: 5 minutes

1. In a medium bowl, combine tuna and seasonings. Mix well.

2. Stir in tomato, onion, and cilantro.

3. Divide mixture between lettuce leaves, and wrap them up.

MAKES 1 SERVING

Turkey Ranch Meatloaf Muffins

1/12 of recipe (1 muffin): 94 calories, 3.5g fat, 180mg sodium, 5g carbs, 0.5g fiber, 2g sugars, 10.5g protein

1¼ pounds raw lean ground turkey (7% fat or less)

½ cup old-fashioned oats

½ cup finely chopped onion

½ cup finely chopped celery

Half of a 1-ounce packet (about 1½ tablespoons) ranch dressing/dip seasoning mix

3 tablespoons egg whites or fat-free liquid egg substitute

¼ cup ketchup

You'll Need: 12-cup muffin pan, nonstick spray, large bowl

Prep: 15 minutes

Cook: 35 minutes

1. Preheat oven to 375 degrees. Spray a 12-cup muffin pan with nonstick spray.

2. In a large bowl, thoroughly mix all ingredients *except* ketchup.

3. Evenly distribute mixture among the muffin cups, and smooth out the tops. Evenly top with ketchup.

4. Bake until firm with lightly browned edges, 30 to 35 minutes.

MAKES 12 SERVINGS

Cheesy Tuna Mushrooms

½ of recipe (1 stuffed mushroom): 96 calories, 1.5g fat, 203mg sodium, 7.5g carbs, 2g fiber, 3g sugars, 12.5g protein

2 portabella mushrooms, stems chopped and reserved

One 2.6-ounce pouch low-sodium tuna packed in water

1 wedge The Laughing Cow Light Creamy Swiss cheese

2 teaspoons Best Foods/ Hellman's Dijonnaise

You'll Need: baking sheet, nonstick spray, medium bowl

Prep: 5 minutes

Cook: 20 minutes

1. Preheat oven to 375 degrees. Spray a baking sheet with nonstick spray.

2. Place mushroom caps on the sheet, rounded sides down. Bake until mostly tender, about 12 minutes. Remove sheet, but leave oven on.

3. Meanwhile, in a medium bowl, combine chopped mushroom stems, tuna, cheese, and Dijonnaise. Stir until thoroughly mixed.

4. Blot away excess moisture from mushroom caps. Divide tuna mixture between the caps.

5. Bake until filling is hot and mushroom caps are tender, about 8 minutes.

MAKES 2 SERVINGS

Spicy Baked Cauliflower Bites

Entire recipe: 100 calories, 3g fat, 212mg sodium, 12.5g carbs, 5.5g fiber, 5.5g sugars, 8g protein

2 cups cauliflower florets

1 teaspoon salt-free seasoning mix

¼ teaspoon garlic powder

¼ teaspoon onion powder

1 tablespoon grated Parmesan cheese

You'll Need: baking sheet, nonstick spray, medium microwave-safe bowl

Prep: 5 minutes

Cook: 20 minutes

1. Preheat oven to 425 degrees. Spray a baking sheet with nonstick spray.

2. Place cauliflower in a medium microwave-safe bowl with 2 tablespoons water. Cover and microwave for 2 minutes, or until slightly softened. Drain excess liquid.

3. Lay cauliflower florets closely together on the sheet. Lightly spray with nonstick spray, and sprinkle with seasonings.

4. Bake until tender, about 15 minutes.

5. Top with Parm.

MAKES 1 SERVING

Snack Sips: Smoothies & More

Raise a glass to these sippable snacks!
And don't miss the breakfast smoothies
on page 63 through page 66!

Tropical Green Smoothie

Entire recipe: 100 calories, <0.5g fat, 45mg sodium, 25g carbs, 3g fiber, 19.5g sugars, 2g protein

1⅔ cups spinach leaves

½ cup light orange juice beverage

½ cup frozen unsweetened mango chunks, partially thawed

1 no-calorie sweetener packet

1 cup crushed ice *or* 5 to 8 ice cubes

You'll Need: blender

Prep: 5 minutes

1. Place all ingredients in a blender, along with ¼ cup water.

2. Blend at high speed until smooth, stopping and stirring if needed.

MAKES 1 SERVING

Melon 'n Mint Smoothie

Entire recipe: 100 calories, 0.5g fat, 29mg sodium, 24.5g carbs, 4g fiber, 18g sugars, 2.5g protein

1 cup chopped cantaloupe

1 cup chopped seedless cucumber

½ cup frozen unsweetened strawberries, partially thawed

8 mint leaves

1 teaspoon lemon juice

1 no-calorie sweetener packet

1 cup crushed ice *or* 5 to 8 ice cubes

You'll Need: blender

Prep: 5 minutes

1. Place all ingredients in a blender, along with ¼ cup water.

2. Blend at high speed until smooth, stopping and stirring if needed.

MAKES 1 SERVING

Peach-Berry Freeze 📷

Entire recipe: 90 calories, 2.5g fat, 8mg sodium, 17g carbs, 3.5g fiber, 13g sugars, 1.5g protein

⅔ cup frozen unsweetened peach slices, partially thawed

⅓ cup frozen unsweetened raspberries, partially thawed

½ cup unsweetened coconut milk beverage

½ cup crushed ice *or* 3 to 4 ice cubes

1 to 2 no-calorie sweetener packets

You'll Need: blender

Prep: 5 minutes

1. In a blender, combine peach slices, raspberries, coconut milk beverage, and ice. Add 1 sweetener packet and ¼ cup water.

2. Blend at high speed until smooth, stopping and stirring if needed.

3. If you like, add the second sweetener packet. Mmmm . . .

MAKES 1 SERVING

No-Cal Sweetener Newsflash!

Packets of calorie-free sweetener come in *so* many varieties, including stevia-based kinds and other all-natural picks. Choose your favorite!

Blended Latte

Entire recipe: 95 calories, 4.5g fat, 85mg sodium, 7.5g carbs, 0.5g fiber, 3.5g sugars, 5g protein

2 teaspoons instant coffee granules

1 to 2 no-calorie sweetener packets

⅔ cup light vanilla soymilk

2 tablespoons half & half

1¼ cups crushed ice *or* 6 to 10 ice cubes

You'll Need: tall glass, blender

Prep: 5 minutes

1. In a tall glass, combine coffee granules with 1 sweetener packet. Add 2 tablespoons hot water, and stir to dissolve.

2. Transfer mixture to a blender. Add soymilk, half & half, and ice. Blend at high speed until smooth.

3. If you like, add the second sweetener packet.

MAKES 1 SERVING

PB Vanilla Protein Shake

Entire recipe: 100 calories, 3.5g fat, 205mg sodium, 7.5g carbs, 1.5g fiber, 1.5g sugars, 11g protein

¾ cup unsweetened vanilla almond milk

2 tablespoons vanilla protein powder with about 100 calories per serving

1½ tablespoons powdered peanut butter

1 no-calorie sweetener packet

1 cup crushed ice *or* 5 to 8 ice cubes

You'll Need: blender

Prep: 5 minutes

Combine all ingredients in a blender, and blend until smooth.

MAKES 1 SERVING

HG FYI

Get the full 411 about powdered peanut butter on page 64!

Easy Hot Cocoa 📷

Entire recipe: 91 calories, 3.5g fat, 71mg sodium, 12g carbs, 3g fiber, 6g sugars, 5.5g protein

1½ tablespoons unsweetened cocoa powder

1 no-calorie sweetener packet

1 teaspoon mini semi-sweet chocolate chips

⅔ cup light vanilla soymilk

You'll Need: microwave-safe mug or glass

Prep: 5 minutes

Cook: 5 minutes or less

1. Place cocoa powder, sweetener, and chocolate chips in a microwave-safe mug or glass. Add ¼ cup very hot water, and stir until mostly dissolved. Add soymilk, and mix well.

2. Microwave until hot, about 1 minute.

MAKES 1 SERVING

Sweet Treats

DESSERT TIME! Whether you're craving creamy peanut butter, tropical fruit, rich chocolate, or sweet apple cinnamon treats . . . This chapter's got you covered!

PB&J Caramel Crunchcake 📷

Entire recipe: 100 calories, 1g fat, 85mg sodium, 18.5g carbs, 1.5g fiber, 8g sugars, 4.5g protein

2 tablespoons fat-free
vanilla yogurt

1 tablespoon powdered
peanut butter

1 caramel rice cake

2 tablespoons chopped
strawberries

You'll Need: small bowl

Prep: 5 minutes

1. In a small bowl, combine yogurt with powdered peanut butter. Stir until uniform.

2. Spread mixture over rice cake, and top with strawberries.

MAKES 1 SERVING

HG FYI

Get the full 411 about powdered peanut butter on page 64!

Fruity Popcorn Crunch

Entire recipe: 100 calories, 0.5g fat, 173mg sodium, 29g carbs, 9.5g fiber, 5.5g sugars, 2g protein

2½ cups popped 94% fat-free microwave popcorn

¼ cup Fiber One Original bran cereal

¼ cup bite-sized freeze-dried fruit (if using large pieces, break them up into smaller pieces)

You'll Need: sealable container

Prep: 5 minutes

Combine all ingredients in a sealable container. Seal and shake.

MAKES 1 SERVING

Churro Chips 'n Dip

Entire recipe: 91 calories, 0.5g fat, 42mg sodium, 18g carbs, 1.5g fiber, 7g sugars, 3.5g protein

One 6-inch corn tortilla

Half of a no-calorie sweetener packet

⅛ teaspoon plus 1 dash cinnamon

¼ cup fat-free vanilla yogurt

You'll Need: baking sheet, nonstick spray, small bowl

Prep: 5 minutes

Cook: 10 minutes

1. Preheat oven to 400 degrees. Spray a baking sheet with nonstick spray.

2. Evenly cut tortilla into six wedges. Lightly spray with nonstick spray. Evenly coat both sides with the sweetener and ⅛ teaspoon cinnamon.

3. Lay wedges close together on the sheet, and bake for 5 minutes.

4. Carefully flip wedges. Bake until crispy, 2 to 4 minutes.

5. Meanwhile in a small bowl, stir remaining dash of cinnamon into yogurt.

6. Serve chips with yogurt for dipping.

MAKES 1 SERVING

Easy Apple Chips

Entire recipe: 96 calories, <0.5g fat, 2mg sodium, 25.5g carbs, 5g fiber, 18.5g sugars, 0.5g protein

1 medium Fuji or Granny
Smith apple

½ teaspoon cinnamon

You'll Need: 2 baking sheets, nonstick spray, large bowl

Prep: 10 minutes

Cook: 1 hour

Cool: 10 minutes

1. Arrange oven racks in the center two positions. Preheat oven to 250 degrees. Spray two baking sheets with nonstick spray.

2. Halve apple lengthwise, and remove the core. Slice as thinly as possible, about ⅛-inch thick.

3. Place apple slices in a large bowl, sprinkle with cinnamon, and toss to coat. Lay slices on the baking sheets, evenly spaced.

4. Bake for 30 minutes.

5. Carefully remove baking sheets, and return them to the oven on the opposite racks.

6. Bake until apple slices are dehydrated and slightly shriveled, about 30 more minutes.

7. Let cool, about 10 minutes.

MAKES 1 SERVING

Grilled Fruit Kebabs

Entire recipe: 96 calories, <0.5g fat, 2mg sodium, 25g carbs, 3g fiber, 20g sugars, 1.5g protein

½ cup 1-inch pineapple chunks

⅓ cup 1-inch mango chunks

⅓ cup 1-inch peach chunks

¼ teaspoon cinnamon

You'll Need: 2 skewers, grill pan, nonstick spray

Prep: 10 minutes

Cook: 10 minutes

1. Alternately thread fruit chunks onto 2 skewers, tightly packing them together. Sprinkle with cinnamon.

2. Bring a grill pan sprayed with nonstick spray to medium-high heat. Cook until fruit is slightly blackened and caramelized, about 8 minutes, rotating to evenly cook.

MAKES 1 SERVING

HG FYI

If using wooden skewers, first soak them in water for about 20 minutes to prevent burning.

Cherry-Good Baked Apple

Entire recipe: 94 calories, <0.5g fat, 18mg sodium, 25g carbs, 4.5g fiber, 18.5g sugars, 0.5g protein

1 medium Rome or Braeburn apple

½ cup zero-calorie cherry soda

⅛ teaspoon cinnamon

You'll Need: loaf pan, nonstick spray

Prep: 5 minutes

Cook: 35 minutes

1. Preheat oven to 375 degrees. Spray a loaf pan with nonstick spray.

2. Halve apple lengthwise, and remove core. Place halves in the pan, cut sides up. Top with soda, and sprinkle with cinnamon.

3. Bake until tender, about 35 minutes.

MAKES 1 SERVING

Microwave Alternative

Place apple halves in a medium microwave-safe bowl. Top with soda, and sprinkle with cinnamon. Cover and microwave for 5 minutes, or until tender.

Sweet 'n Spiced Baked Pear

Entire recipe: 90 calories, <0.5g fat, 82mg sodium, 23g carbs, 4.5g fiber, 14.5g sugars, 0.5g protein

1 small pear (Bosc pears work great)

½ cup zero-calorie cream soda

⅛ teaspoon cinnamon

You'll Need: loaf pan, nonstick spray

Prep: 5 minutes

Cook: 35 minutes

1. Preheat oven to 375 degrees. Spray a loaf pan with nonstick spray.

2. Halve pear lengthwise, and remove core. Place halves in the pan, cut sides up. Top with soda, and sprinkle with cinnamon.

3. Bake until tender, about 35 minutes.

MAKES 1 SERVING

Microwave Alternative

Place pear halves in a medium microwave-safe bowl, cut sides up. Top with soda, and sprinkle with cinnamon. Cover and microwave for 5 minutes, or until tender.

Apple Cinnamon Ricotta Bowl

Entire recipe: 94 calories, 2.5g fat, 84mg sodium, 12.5g carbs, 2g fiber, 9.5g sugars, 6g protein

¼ **cup light/low-fat ricotta cheese**

Half of a no-calorie sweetener packet

1 drop vanilla extract

⅛ **teaspoon plus 1 dash cinnamon**

½ **cup chopped apple**

You'll Need: medium bowl

Prep: 5 minutes

1. In a medium bowl, combine ricotta cheese, sweetener, vanilla extract, and ⅛ teaspoon cinnamon. Mix well.

2. Top with apple, and sprinkle with remaining dash of cinnamon.

MAKES 1 SERVING

Berries 'n Cream Bowl

Entire recipe: 100 calories, 3.5g fat, 83mg sodium, 13g carbs, 4g fiber, 7.5g sugars, 6.5g protein

¼ cup light/low-fat ricotta cheese

1 drop vanilla extract

1 no-calorie sweetener packet

½ cup raspberries and/or blackberries

½ teaspoon mini semi-sweet chocolate chips

You'll Need: medium bowl

Prep: 5 minutes

1. In a medium bowl, combine ricotta, vanilla extract, and sweetener. Mix well.

2. Top with berries, and sprinkle with chocolate chips.

MAKES 1 SERVING

Supreme Fruit Salad

Entire recipe: 99 calories, <0.5g fat, 24mg sodium, 19g carbs, 3.5g fiber, 13g sugars, 6.5g protein

¼ cup fat-free plain Greek yogurt

1 drop vanilla extract

Half of a no-calorie sweetener packet

Dash cinnamon

½ cup chopped strawberries

¼ cup chopped apple

¼ cup blueberries

You'll Need: medium bowl

Prep: 5 minutes

1. In a medium bowl, combine yogurt, vanilla extract, sweetener, and cinnamon. Mix well.

2. Add fruit, and stir to coat.

MAKES 1 SERVING

Lemon Blueberry Crepe

Entire recipe: 100 calories, 0.5g fat, 134mg sodium, 13g carbs, 1.5g fiber, 9.5g sugars, 12g protein

¼ cup egg whites

2 teaspoons vanilla protein powder with about 100 calories per serving

2 dashes cinnamon

⅓ cup blueberries

3 tablespoons fat-free lemon yogurt (or fat-free vanilla yogurt with three drops of lemon juice)

HG FYI

Flip to page 80 for crepe tips 'n tricks!

You'll Need: 2 small bowls, whisk, 10-inch skillet, nonstick spray, offset spatula or flexible rubber spatula, plate

Prep: 5 minutes

Cook: 5 minutes

1. To make the batter, in a small bowl, combine egg whites, protein powder, and cinnamon. Whisk until uniform.

2. To make the crepe, bring a 10-inch skillet sprayed with nonstick spray to medium heat. Pour batter into the pan, quickly tilting the skillet in all directions to evenly coat the bottom. Cook until lightly browned on the bottom, about 2 minutes. Carefully flip with an offset spatula or flexible rubber spatula. Cook until lightly browned on the other side, about 1 minute.

3. Transfer the crepe to a plate.

4. In another small bowl, combine blueberries with yogurt, and stir to coat. Place mixture in the center of the crepe, and wrap crepe around the filling.

MAKES 1 SERVING

Apple Cinnamon Wonton Cups

⅓ of recipe (2 wonton cups): 93 calories, <0.5g fat, 81mg sodium, 19g carbs, 1.5g fiber, 9.5g sugars, 3.5g protein

6 small square wonton wrappers

1¼ cups chopped Fuji apple (or another sweet apple)

1½ teaspoons brown sugar (not packed)

¼ teaspoon cinnamon

¼ cup plus 2 tablespoons fat-free vanilla Greek yogurt

HG Tip!

Store extra wonton cups at room temperature in a sealed bag or container. Store apple mixture and yogurt in sealed containers in the fridge.

You'll Need: 6-cup or 12-cup muffin pan, nonstick spray, medium-large microwave-safe bowl

Prep: 10 minutes

Cook: 10 minutes

Cool: 10 minutes

1. Preheat oven to 350 degrees. Spray a 6-cup muffin pan (or half a 12-cup pan) with nonstick spray.

2. Place each wonton wrapper in a sprayed cup of the muffin pan; press it into the bottom and sides. Lightly spray with nonstick spray. Bake until lightly browned, about 8 minutes.

3. Let cool completely, about 10 minutes.

4. In a medium-large microwave-safe bowl, mix apples with sugar and cinnamon. Cover and microwave until apples have softened, about 2 minutes.

5. Just before eating, divide ⅓ of apple mixture (about ¼ cup) between 2 wonton cups. Top each wonton cup with 1 tablespoon yogurt.

MAKES 3 SERVINGS

Tropical Fruit Fillo Shells

⅓ of recipe (5 shells): 100 calories, 4g fat, 54mg sodium, 16g carbs, 0.5g fiber, 4.5g sugars, 2.5g protein

15 frozen mini fillo shells

1 tablespoon white chocolate chips, finely chopped

¼ cup finely chopped peaches (fresh or thawed from frozen)

1 tablespoon shredded sweetened coconut, chopped

You'll Need: baking sheet

Prep: 5 minutes

Cook: 5 minutes

1. Preheat oven to 350 degrees.

2. Place shells on a baking sheet. Evenly distribute chopped white chocolate chips among the shells.

3. Bake until chopped chips have softened, about 5 minutes.

4. Evenly distribute peaches and chopped coconut among the shells.

MAKES 3 SERVINGS

For the latest food news, recipes, tips 'n tricks, and more, **sign up for free daily emails at hungry-girl.com!**

Cannoli Fillo Shells

⅓ of recipe (5 shells): 100 calories, 4g fat, 78mg sodium, 14g carbs, <0.5g fiber, 2.5g sugars, 5g protein

15 frozen mini fillo shells

⅓ cup light/low-fat ricotta cheese

⅛ teaspoon vanilla extract

1 no-calorie sweetener packet

1½ teaspoons mini semi-sweet chocolate chips

You'll Need: baking sheet, medium bowl

Prep: 5 minutes

Cook: 5 minutes

1. Preheat oven to 350 degrees.

2. Place shells on a baking sheet, and bake until lightly browned and crispy, 3 to 5 minutes.

3. In a medium bowl, combine ricotta cheese, vanilla extract, and sweetener. Mix well.

4. Just before eating, evenly distribute ⅓ of the ricotta mixture (about 1½ tablespoons) among 5 shells, and top with ½ teaspoon chocolate chips.

MAKES 3 SERVINGS

HG Tip!

Store extra fillo shells at room temperature in a sealed bag or container. Store ricotta mixture in a sealed container in the fridge.

Open-Faced S'mores

Entire recipe: 99 calories, 2g fat, 81mg sodium, 19g carbs, 1g fiber, 10g sugars, 1g protein

3 low-fat honey graham crackers (¾ths of a sheet)

15 mini marshmallows

1 teaspoon mini chocolate chips

You'll Need: baking sheet

Prep: 5 minutes

Cook: 5 minutes or less

1. Preheat broiler (or preheat oven to 500 degrees).

2. Lay crackers on a baking sheet. Evenly top with marshmallows and chocolate chips.

3. Broil until marshmallows have browned and chocolate chips have melted, 1 to 2 minutes.

MAKES 1 SERVING

Microwave Alternative

Lay crackers on a microwave-safe plate. Evenly top with marshmallows and chocolate chips. Microwave for 30 seconds, or until marshmallows and chocolate chips have melted.

Chocolate-Drizzled Raspberries

Entire recipe: 96 calories, 3g fat, 4mg sodium, 17g carbs, 6.5g fiber, 9.5g sugars, 1.5g protein

¾ cup raspberries

2 teaspoons mini semi-sweet chocolate chips

1 teaspoon fat-free milk, light vanilla soymilk, or unsweetened vanilla almond milk

You'll Need: medium bowl, very small microwave-safe bowl

Prep: 5 minutes

Cook: 5 minutes or less

1. Place raspberries in a medium bowl.

2. In a very small microwave-safe bowl, combine chocolate chips with milk. Microwave at 50 percent power for 25 seconds.

3. Stir until smooth and uniform. Drizzle over raspberries.

4. Enjoy immediately, or refrigerate until chocolate drizzle is firm.

MAKES 1 SERVING

HG Alternative

Try this recipe with 50 calories' worth of any fruit—see the fruit chart on page 341!

Freeze! Brownie Storing Tips 'n Tricks

Unless you've got 23 friends over, chances are you're going to want to freeze some of those leftover brownies! Here's the need-to-know . . .

To Freeze . . . Tightly wrap each cooled brownie in plastic wrap. Place individually wrapped brownies in sealable containers, seal, and place in the freezer.

To Thaw . . . Unwrap a brownie, and place on a microwave-safe plate. Microwave at 50 percent power for 30 seconds, or until it reaches your desired temperature.

Double-Chocolate Brownie Bites 📷

¼₄ of recipe (one 2-inch brownie): 94 calories, 2g fat, 169mg sodium, 18.5g carbs, 1.5g fiber, 10.5g sugars, 1g protein

1 box moist-style devil's food cake mix (15.25 to 18.25 ounces)

One 15-ounce can pure pumpkin

¼ cup mini semi-sweet chocolate chips

You'll Need: 9-inch by 13-inch baking pan, nonstick spray, large bowl

Prep: 10 minutes

Cook: 30 minutes

1. Preheat oven to 400 degrees. Spray a 9-inch by 13-inch baking pan with nonstick spray.

2. In a large bowl, mix cake mix with pumpkin until completely smooth and uniform. (Batter will be thick.)

3. Spread mixture into the baking pan. Evenly top with chocolate chips and lightly press into the batter.

4. Bake until a toothpick inserted into the center comes out mostly clean, 25 to 30 minutes.

5. Let brownies cool. Slice lengthwise into fourths, and slice widthwise into sixths.

MAKES 24 SERVINGS

Protein-Packed Chocolate Cake in a Mug

Entire recipe: 97 calories, 3g fat, 230mg sodium, 9.5g carbs, 4.5g fiber, 2.5g sugars, 9g protein

1 tablespoon coconut flour

1 tablespoon chocolate protein powder with about 100 calories per serving

½ tablespoon unsweetened cocoa powder

¼ teaspoon baking powder

Half of a no-calorie sweetener packet

2 tablespoons egg whites or fat-free liquid egg substitute

3 tablespoons unsweetened vanilla almond milk

⅛ teaspoon vanilla extract

½ teaspoon mini semi-sweet chocolate chips

You'll Need: microwave-safe mug, nonstick spray

Prep: 5 minutes

Cook: 5 minutes or less

1. Spray a microwave-safe mug with nonstick spray. Add flour, protein powder, cocoa powder, baking powder, and sweetener. Mix well.

2. Add egg whites/substitute, 1 tablespoon almond milk, vanilla extract, and 2 tablespoons water. Stir until uniform.

3. Microwave for 1 minute and 15 seconds, or until set.

4. Sprinkle with chocolate chips, and drizzle with remaining 2 tablespoons almond milk. Eat warm.

MAKES 1 SERVING

Photo Alert!

The camera icon next to the recipe name means flip to the insert to see a photo of this recipe. Find full-color photos of ALL the recipes at hungry-girl.com/books.

Blueberry Lemon Super Muffins 📷

⅙ of recipe (1 muffin): 98 calories, 1.5g fat, 206mg sodium, 15.5g carbs, 3g fiber, 8g sugars, 5.5g protein

¼ cup coconut flour

¼ cup whole-wheat flour

3 tablespoons granulated white sugar

¼ teaspoon salt

⅛ teaspoon baking soda

¾ cup egg whites or fat-free liquid egg substitute

3 tablespoons fat-free plain Greek yogurt

1½ tablespoons lemon juice

1 tablespoon light whipped butter or light buttery spread, room temperature

¾ teaspoon lemon zest

⅛ teaspoon vanilla extract

½ cup frozen unsweetened blueberries

You'll Need: 6-cup or 12-cup muffin pan, nonstick spray, medium bowl, large bowl, whisk

Prep: 15 minutes

Cook: 25 minutes

1. Preheat oven to 350 degrees. Spray a 6-cup muffin pan (or half a 12-cup pan) with nonstick spray.

2. In a medium bowl, combine both flours, sugar, salt, and baking soda. Mix well.

3. In a large bowl, combine egg whites/substitute, yogurt, lemon juice, butter, lemon zest, and vanilla extract. Whisk until thoroughly blended. (Don't worry if butter bits do not break up completely.)

4. Add flour mixture to the large bowl. Mix until uniform. Fold in blueberries.

5. Evenly distribute batter among the 6 sprayed cups of the muffin pan.

6. Bake until a toothpick inserted into the center of a muffin comes out clean, about 25 minutes.

MAKES 6 SERVINGS

Freeze! Muffin Storing Tips 'n Tricks

Wanna save leftover muffins in the freezer? Read up!

To Freeze . . . Tightly wrap each cooled muffin in plastic wrap. Place individually wrapped muffins in sealable containers, seal, and place in the freezer.

To Thaw . . . Unwrap a muffin, and place on a microwave-safe plate. Microwave at 50 percent power for 30 seconds, or until it reaches your desired temperature.

Apple Cinnamon Super Muffins

⅙ of recipe (1 muffin): 97 calories, 1.5g fat, 206mg sodium, 15g carbs, 3g fiber, 8g sugars, 5.5g protein

¼ cup coconut flour

¼ cup whole-wheat flour

3 tablespoons granulated sugar

¼ teaspoon salt

¼ teaspoon cinnamon

⅛ teaspoon baking soda

¾ cup egg whites or fat-free liquid egg substitute

3 tablespoons fat-free plain Greek yogurt

1 tablespoon light whipped butter or light buttery spread, room temperature

½ teaspoon vanilla extract

½ cup peeled and chopped Fuji apple (or another sweet apple)

You'll Need: 6-cup or 12-cup muffin pan, nonstick spray, medium bowl, large bowl, whisk

Prep: 15 minutes

Cook: 25 minutes

1. Preheat oven to 350 degrees. Spray a 6-cup muffin pan (or half a 12-cup pan) with nonstick spray.

2. In a medium bowl, combine both flours, sugar, salt, cinnamon, and baking soda. Mix well.

3. In a large bowl, combine egg whites/substitute, yogurt, butter, and vanilla extract. Whisk until thoroughly blended. (Don't worry if butter bits do not break up completely.)

4. Add flour mixture to the large bowl. Mix until uniform. Fold in apples.

5. Evenly distribute batter among the 6 sprayed cups of the muffin pan.

6. Bake until a toothpick inserted into the center of a muffin comes out clean, about 22 minutes.

MAKES 6 SERVINGS

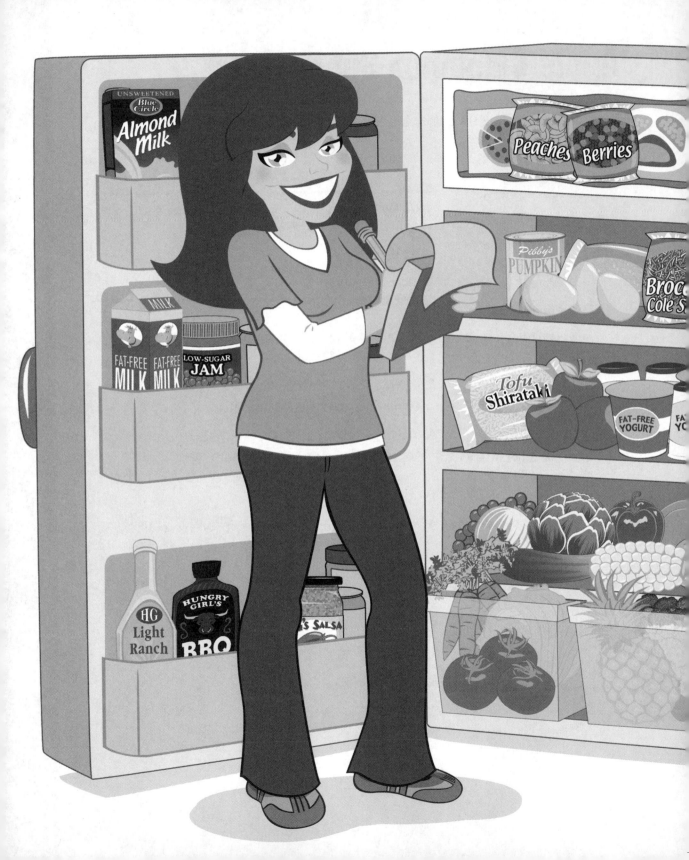

GO-TO GUIDE FOR GROCERY SHOPPING, MONEY SAVING, MEAL PREPPING & MORE

Supermarket List

Here are some staples to stock up on, plus helpful tips and brands we love . . .

DAIRY/REFRIGERATED

Cheese

The Laughing Cow Light Creamy Swiss cheese

Sargento Reduced Fat sliced cheese

> *Sargento's cheese slices are lower in sodium than most brands.*

Shredded reduced-fat cheddar and Mexican-blend cheese

Shredded part-skim mozzarella cheese

Crumbled reduced-fat feta cheese

Light/low-fat ricotta cheese

> *Don't confuse this with part-skim ricotta, which has significantly more calories and fat!*

Grated Parmesan cheese

Yogurt

Fat-free plain and vanilla Greek yogurt

> ➤ Fage Total 0%, Chobani 0%, Oikos 0%, Yoplait Greek 100, Dannon Light & Fit Greek

Fat-free vanilla yogurt

> ➤ Yoplait Light, Dannon Light & Fit

Egg Products

Fat-free liquid egg substitute

> ➤ Egg Beaters Original, Better'n Eggs, Nulaid ReddiEgg

Liquid egg whites

> ➤ AllWhites, Egg Beaters 100% Egg Whites

Large whole eggs

Milk

Fat-free milk

Dairy milk is a must for several of the breakfast recipes, due to its impressively high protein count. Choose lactose-free, if needed, or look for a milk swap with added protein.

Other Refrigerated Staples

Light whipped butter or light buttery spread

Look for those with 50 calories or less and around 5g fat per tablespoon.

> ➤ Brummel & Brown, Land O' Lakes, Smart Balance

Light sour cream

House Foods Tofu Shirataki Noodle Substitute

Find this low-calorie pasta swap near the tofu. Don't confuse it with plain shirataki noodles, which don't taste as good!

PANTRY

Canned/Jarred Foods

Canned pure pumpkin

> *Not pumpkin pie filling—that has twice as many calories and four times as much sugar!*
>
> ➤ Libby's 100%

Canned beans: black, garbanzo/chickpeas, kidney beans

Canned crushed tomatoes

Salsa or pico de gallo with 90mg sodium or less per 2-tablespoon serving (refrigerated and shelf-stable)

Cereal

Fiber One Original bran cereal

> *Avoiding aspartame? Go with All-Bran Original or Nature's Path Organic SmartBran cereal.*

Old-fashioned oats

> *Not instant or five-minute oats . . . These slow-cooking oats are a must!*
>
> ➤ Quaker

Sauces, Seasonings, and Shelf-Stable Staples

BBQ sauce with 45 calories or less per 2-tablespoon serving

Sauces and marinades with 25 calories or less per tablespoon

> ➤ Lawry's, Margie's, Ken's, Mrs. Dash, Newman's Own

Salad dressings with 25 calories or less per tablespoon

> ➤ Newman's Own Lite, Ken's Light Options, Kraft Lite, Wish-Bone Light

Olive oil, extra-virgin olive oil, and/or grapeseed oil

Grapeseed oil is super versatile with a mild taste . . .
Try it!

Vinegar (balsamic, red wine, white wine, rice, or cider)

Low-sugar preserves

➤ Smuckers

Creamy peanut butter

Powdered peanut butter

Only about 45 calories and 1.5 grams of fat per 2-tablespoon
serving! Worth ordering online.

➤ PB2, FitNutz, Just Great Stuff

Light mayonnaise

Salt-free seasoning mix

➤ Mrs. Dash

Ranch dressing/dip seasoning mix

Taco seasoning mix

No-calorie sweetener packets

Choose your favorite type . . . There are many natural
options on shelves!

➤ Truvia, Splenda, Stevia in the Raw,
   Monk Fruit in the Raw

Vanilla protein powder with about 100 calories per serving

➤ Designer Whey, Rainbow Light, Quest,
   Jay Robb, Tera's Whey

Nuts

Pistachios in the shell

> ➤ Everybody's Nuts!, Wonderful Pistachios

Almonds (whole and sliced)

> ➤ Blue Diamond, Emerald, Wonderful (whole nuts and Almond Accents)

Chopped walnuts

Breads

100-calorie flat sandwich buns

> ➤ Flatout Foldits (Hungry Girl varieties and others!), Arnold/Brownberry/Oroweat Sandwich Thins, Pepperidge Farm Deli Flats, Nature's Own Sandwich Rounds

Light English muffins

> ➤ Thomas', Western Bagel Alternative, Fiber One

Light bread slices (45 calories or less per slice)

> ➤ Nature's Own 40 Calories, Nature's Own Double Fiber, Arnold/Brownberry, Sara Lee 45 Calories & Delightful, Pepperidge Farm Light Style, Pepperidge Farm Very Thin, Fiber One

Medium-large high-fiber flour tortillas with 110 calories or less

> ➤ La Tortilla Factory

6-inch corn tortillas

> ➤ Mission

MEAT AND SEAFOOD

Meat and Meat Swaps

Boneless skinless chicken breast (raw and/or precooked)

No-salt-added turkey breast

> *Check the deli counter! Can't find it? Just get the turkey with the lowest sodium count you see.*
>
> ➤ Boar's Head

Extra-lean ground beef (4% fat or less; at least 96% lean)

Lean ground turkey (7% fat or less; at least 93% lean)

Frozen ground-beef-style soy crumbles

> ➤ MorningStar Farms Meal Starters Grillers Recipe Crumbles, Boca Veggie Ground Crumbles

Seafood

Canned and pouched low-sodium tuna packed in water

> ➤ StarKist

Raw large shrimp

Ready-to-eat shrimp

Raw tilapia, cod, or sea bass

PRODUCE

Check out the seasonal produce guide on page 313!

Fresh Vegetables

High-fiber veggies (tomatoes, onions, bell peppers, green beans, sugar snap peas, snow peas, bean sprouts, broccoli, Brussels sprouts, carrots, jicama)

High-volume veggies (mushrooms, cucumbers, cabbage, celery, zucchini, eggplant, yellow squash, asparagus, cauliflower, kale, spinach)

Romaine or iceberg lettuce

Spaghetti squash

Bagged Produce

Lettuce mixes

Broccoli cole slaw

Frozen Vegetables

High-fiber veggies (peppers, green beans, sugar snap peas, snow peas, broccoli, Brussels sprouts, carrots)

High-volume veggies (mushrooms, asparagus, cauliflower, kale)

Sweet corn kernels

Cauliflower florets

Fresh Fruit

Apples

Bananas

Blueberries

Raspberries and/or blackberries

Strawberries

Plus, choose your favorites from page 341!

Frozen Fruit (No Sugar Added)

Blackberries

Blueberries

Mango

Peach slices

Raspberries

Strawberries

Seasonal Produce Guide

Whipping up meals and snacks with seasonal fruits and veggies is great for two reasons:

1. Produce that's at its peak freshness tastes fantastic.

2. When there's an abundance of produce (which is usually the case with seasonal selections), grocery stores tend to lower costs to sell it all while it's still fresh.

Double win! Read on, and stock up according to season . . .

Spring

Asparagus	Snap peas	Oranges
Spinach	Strawberries	Green beans
Mangoes		

Summer

Cucumbers	Summer squash	Cherries
Eggplant	Tomatoes	Melons (most varieties)
Green beans	Berries (most varieties)	Peaches/Nectarines

Fall

Broccoli	Butternut squash	Pears
Brussels sprouts	Spaghetti squash	Pomegranates
Cauliflower	Grapes	

Winter

Brussels sprouts	Spaghetti squash	Pears
Butternut squash	Oranges (most varieties)	Pomegranates
Kale	Grapefruit	

Year-Round

Bell peppers	Broccoli	Apples
Cabbage	Lettuce	Avocados
Carrots	Mushrooms	Bananas

Budget-Friendly Grocery Guide

It's totally possible to eat smart and lose weight without spending a lot of money. Here are some cash-saving tips 'n tricks . . .

Buy shelf-stable staples in bulk

Purchase the jumbo-sized containers, and stock up when there's a sale. Old-fashioned oats, almonds, canned goods (pure pumpkin, beans, canned crushed tomatoes, etc.) . . . Fill your pantry!

Shop store brands

While the supermarket list on the previous pages calls out some brand-name superstars, you can save big bucks buying generic products. These days, many are nearly identical to the big-brand items. Some generic Hungryland staples? Fat-free milk, light sour cream, canned beans, crushed tomatoes, light mayo, and frozen fruits and veggies.

Become a coupon queen

It's nothing groundbreaking, but it works. (There's a reason extreme couponing is a thing!) Scour the Sunday paper, get a grocery-store discount card, and frequent online coupon websites; some of those sites will apply savings right to your supermarket card!

Utilize leftover ingredients

If you crack open a can of black beans for a stir-fry, don't let the rest go to waste. Flip to the index, and find more black-bean recipes to make!

Shop seasonally

Produce is freshest and least expensive when it's in season. So bake spaghetti-squash dishes in winter, and whip up berry bowls in summer! And when a recipe calls for your choice of high-fiber veggies, high-volume veggies, and 50 or 100 calories' worth of fruit, head straight for the seasonal picks . . . Check out the guide on pages 313 to 314!

Prep it yourself

Precut vegetables are convenient, but they're also pricier. Save cash by buying heads of lettuce, whole broccoli, stem-on green beans, and more.

Hit the freezer aisle

Fish, shrimp, fruits, veggies . . . Frozen varieties are often available at lower costs, and they're just as nutritious. Check the ingredient lists to make sure nothing's been added, like salt or sweeteners.

Check out the meat and seafood counters

Not only can you find more options, but you'll also be able to buy the exact amount you need.

Time-Saving Tips & Plan-Ahead Ideas: Veggies

Buy 'em frozen

You'll save the time you'd spend cutting *and* cooking, since freezer-aisle veggies are usually precut and precooked. Just thaw or nuke, and add to your dish when the raw veggies would have just a minute or two left of cook time.

Look for . . . bell peppers, onions, green beans, sugar snap peas, snow peas, bean sprouts, broccoli, Brussels sprouts, carrots, mushrooms, zucchini, yellow squash, asparagus, cauliflower, and kale.

Check out canned options

Canned veggies can get a bad rap, but they're not bad in a pinch. Like frozen types, they're precut and precooked. Add 'em to your recipe with just enough time to heat.

Look for . . . tomatoes, green beans, carrots, mushrooms, and asparagus.

Label warning!

Frozen and canned veggies can contain added salt, which will alter the sodium count of a recipe calling for fresh. Read the ingredient lists, and look for cans labeled "no salt added."

Hit the fridge

Prewashed, precut bagged produce is a lifesaver for time-crunched dieters. Some packages are even designed to let you steam the veggies right in the bag!

> **Look for . . .** onions, bell peppers, kale, spinach, and bagged lettuce mixes. In a pinch, hit the supermarket salad bar!

Budget tip!

Have a little time to spare on the weekend, but not so much on busy weekdays? Buy whole veggies—which are cheaper than the precut kinds—and devote some time on Sunday to getting them in ready-to-eat-or-cook shape. Stash them in sealable containers or storage bags; then when the time comes, you'll be ready to go!

Time-Saving Tips & Plan-Ahead Ideas: Chicken

Whether a recipe calls for raw or cooked chicken, you can buy it precooked—the less sodium the better. Look for fresh or frozen strips, cutlets, and chopped chicken. You can also cook up a big batch ahead of time—check out the easy how-to below. And here's a handy raw-to-cooked conversion guideline: When substituting cooked chicken for raw, use ¾ of the raw amount. So if a recipe calls for 4 ounces raw chicken, use 3 ounces cooked.

How to Cook Chicken à la HG . . .

Place raw boneless skinless chicken breast on a baking sheet sprayed with nonstick spray, and sprinkle with salt-free seasoning mix. Bake at 375 degrees until cooked through, about 20 minutes. (Cook time will be longer for large batches.) Voilá!

P.S. For perfectly cooked chicken, use a food thermometer, and bake until the internal temperature is 165 degrees.

Skillet Alternative: Pound chicken to ½-inch thickness. Bring a skillet sprayed with nonstick spray to medium heat. Cook chicken for about 5 minutes per side, until cooked through. Sprinkle with salt-free seasoning mix.

Time-Saving Tips & Plan-Ahead Ideas: Ground Meat

Many of the ground-meat recipes in this book call for 4 ounces of raw meat. When you buy it by the pound, freeze leftovers in individual 4-ounce portions. Then just thaw in the microwave or fridge before using!

You can also cook the entire batch ahead of time, and freeze in individual portions. Just bring a large skillet sprayed with nonstick spray to medium-high heat. Add beef, and sprinkle with salt-free seasonings. Cook, stir, and crumble until fully cooked, about 10 minutes. Once cool, divide and freeze: 3 ounces of cooked meat is equal to 4 ounces raw.

Rather not freeze your meat, but want to make use of the entire package? Flip to the index, and look up "beef" or "turkey" for more recipes to whip up!

Time-Saving Tips & Plan-Ahead Ideas: Eggs

Hard-boiled egg whites are called for in lots of Hungry Girl Diet meals. (They also make a great snack—have FIVE for about 85 calories!) So don't wait until you're whipping up an oatmeal breakfast to boil those eggs. Hard-boil a dozen eggs in advance, so you don't have to scramble (no pun intended) once mealtime rolls around.

Hard-Boil Egg Whites in Four Fast Steps. . .

1. Place eggs in a pot, and cover completely with hot water, leaving a few inches of the pot's inner edge above the water line.

2. Bring to a boil, and cook for 10 minutes.

3. Drain water, and fill the pot with very cold water. (Add ice, if you have it.)

4. Once cool, peel off the shells, slice in half, and remove the yolks.

Super Swaps for Hard-Boiled Egg Whites

"HG, I forgot to hard-boil those eggs/I don't like hard-boiled eggs/
I just want some other options!" We've got you covered with these
alternatives . . .

Protein Powder: If you're making a hot cereal breakfast, start by
adding two tablespoons of protein powder to the water (make
sure it's cold); stir to dissolve. Then add the water to the pot where
directed.

Egg Scramble: Cook egg whites (or egg substitute) with nonstick
spray in a skillet or in a microwave-safe mug in the microwave; add
salt-free seasonings to taste. Those 2 large egg whites are equal to
about ¼ cup liquid egg whites or fat-free liquid egg substitute.

Chicken: Got some cooked skinless chicken breast chillin' in
the fridge? Snack on an ounce of it in place of 2 egg whites—
practically the same number of calories and grams of protein!

Hot Cereal Super-Sizer: Stir ¼ cup liquid egg whites or fat-free
liquid egg substitute into your oatmeal or oat bran while it cooks.
Add it just after you reduce to a simmer. The result will be a larger
(and creamier) bowl of cereal, and it'll taste great!

Meal Freezing DOs and DON'Ts

Want to prep your food ahead of time, and keep a freezer full of healthy meals? Do it! Just follow this advice . . .

DO let your food cool completely before freezing it. Otherwise, it could lower the temperature of your freezer and affect the foods around it.

DON'T freeze your meal in a container that isn't meant for the microwave. Use a sealable plastic container with a lid—one that's labeled microwave safe.

DO freeze breakfast sandwiches, hot cereal, stir-frys, and foil packs. Just don't nuke those packs *in* the foil!

DON'T freeze shirataki or veggie dishes with a high water content. Lettuce, cucumbers, zucchini, spaghetti squash . . . These won't fare well upon thawing.

DO lay a piece of plastic wrap directly on the food's surface before freezing it. This will limit the formation of ice crystals and help maintain your food's texture. Just remember to remove it before you reheat.

Ready to reheat?

Pop the lid to vent, and microwave for 2 minutes at a time, stopping and stirring. As for those breakfast sandwiches, wrap them in paper towels, and cook at 50 percent power for 1 minute; then cook on full power for 15 seconds, or until hot.

Multiply Your Meals: Turn Single-Serving Recipes into Family-Friendly Dishes

Double or quadruple recipes with ease . . . Here are some tips 'n tricks!

Go up a size or two in cookware

If the recipe calls for a basic skillet, you'll probably need a large or extra-large one. If a small pot is called for, use a medium or large one. You get the picture!

Find the correct cook time by paying attention to recipe cues

This isn't an exact science—you can't always just double or quadruple the time—which is why indicators are so helpful. Keep a close eye on the appearance of your food as you cook it. The recipes in this book will tell you if the veggies should be slightly softened or fully softened, if the cooking liquid should be thickened or absorbed, etc. These cues will guide you to the appropriate cook times.

Increase seasonings to taste

You don't always need to fully multiply herbs and spices; they can become overpowering. Try starting with the original amount, and then add more to taste as you go!

Pssst . . . Don't miss these multi-serving meals!

LUNCH & DINNER

Big Beef Skillet (page 100)

Upside-Down Shepherd's Pie (page 101)

Butternut Squash & Chicken Sausage Skillet (page 105)

Cioppino à la HG (page 130)

Chicken Noodle Bowl (page 132)

Mac 'n Chicken 'n Cheese (page 184)

Shrimp & Pasta Primavera (page 186)

Chicken Pesto Bowl (page 187)

Spaghetti Squash Chicken Girlfredo (page 202)

Spaghetti Squash Bolognese (page 204)

Chicken Cacciatore 'n Spaghetti Squash (page 206)

Spaghetti Squash with Meatballs (page 208)

Meatloaf 'n Mashies (page 226)

SNACKS

Packed-Lunch Pointers

A diet-friendly lunch on the go? Yup!

First and foremost

Pick up an insulated lunch bag—this way, your food will stay cool during your commute. Refrigerate it once you get to the office, if you can. If you don't have access to a fridge, keep a heavy-duty ice pack with your lunch.

Packing a sandwich

Lightly toast the bread to avoid sogginess, and pack high-moisture ingredients (like tomato slices and tuna salad) separately from the bread. Then assemble just before you eat.

Packing a salad

Get yourself a nice big sealable container, plus a small one for salad dressing. Put all your salad fixins in the big container, with the dressing in its own little container. Store the dressing container right inside the large one!

Packing a hot meal

Prep your meal the night before, let it cool, and refrigerate in a sealed microwave-safe container. Once at work, just heat 'n eat . . . or have it chilled. (Cold stir-frys aren't a bad thing!)

A Vegetarian Guide to The Hungry Girl Diet

Meatless Meals & Snacks

Not a meat eater? Check out these no-meat recipes...

BREAKFASTS

Double-Cheese Veggie EggaMuffin *with berries* (page 17)

Guac 'n Veggie B-fast Tostada *with fruit* (page 20)

Over-Medium Egg Sandwich *with fruit* (page 24)

Open-Faced Avocado EggaMuffin *with fruit* (page 27)

Black Bean 'n Cheese Egg Mug *with bun and fruit* (page 28)

Open-Faced Caprese EggaMuffin *with strawberries* (page 29)

Cheesed-Up Spinach B-fast Tostada *with orange segments* (page 30)

Half 'n Half Scramble *with fruit* (page 32)

Breakfast Soft Tacos (page 33)

Open-Faced Poached EggaMuffin *with fruit* (page 34)

Portabella Poached Egg *with fruit-topped yogurt* (page 36)

Strawberry Stuffed Omelette *with PB-topped English muffin* (page 38)

And find more in the pages of *The Hungry Girl Diet*!

Meatless Alternatives

Looking to make some of the meals in this book veggie friendly? It can be done! Specific brands are called out below for fantastic flavor and nutritional stats . . .

Instead of chicken . . .

Find faux-chicken products with 140 calories or less per 4-ounce serving. They come refrigerated and frozen, as both patties and strips. Look for the options with the most protein and the least amount of sodium. Just heat it up (if needed) and add to the rest of the dish.

HG Picks:

➤ MorningStar Farms Grillers Chik'n Veggie Patties (use 1½ patties for every 4 ounces cooked chicken)

➤ Lightlife Smart Strips Chick'n (use 4 ounces for every 4 ounces cooked chicken)

➤ Beyond Meat Chicken-Free Strips (use 3 ounces for every 4 ounces cooked chicken)

Instead of ground beef . . .

I'm all about frozen ground-beef-style soy crumbles! One cup of them is a good alternative to 4 to 5 ounces of raw ground beef or turkey. If a recipe calls for ground meat in order to make a burger, you're better off using a hamburger-style meatless patty with less than 150 calories and 5 grams of fat or less—the more protein, the better.

HG Picks:

➤ MorningStar Farms Meal Starters Grillers Recipe Crumbles

- Boca Ground Crumbles (Note: These are higher in sodium.)

- Gardein The Ultimate Beefless Burger

Need-to-Know Sodium Info

Meat alternatives like the ones mentioned above have more sodium than their meaty counterparts. So if you're swapping, you'll want to skim salt from other places. A few tips to balance out your day . . .

- Since most of these breakfasts are veggie friendly, stick with the options with the lowest sodium content.

- When you pick your snacks, choose those with little to no added salt.

- If the meal you're making calls for any added salt, nix it.

- When choosing a meat-based meal to makeover, opt for one with a low-end sodium count to start with.

HG's Fruit Charts

Use these in recipes that call for your choice of 50 or 100 calories' worth of fruit . . . or just have a 100-calorie portion as a snack! And see the Seasonal Produce Guide on page 313 for the best picks . . .

50-Calorie Portions

1 cup chopped watermelon (0.5g fiber)

1 cup halved strawberries; about 9 large strawberries (3g fiber)

1 cup sliced apple (2.5g fiber)

1 cup chopped cantaloupe (1.5g fiber)

¾ cup blackberries (5.5g fiber)

¾ cup sliced peach; about 1 small peach (1.5g fiber)

¾ cup chopped honeydew melon (1g fiber)

¾ cup raspberries (6g fiber)

¾ cup sliced nectarine; about 1 medium nectarine (2g fiber)

⅔ cup sliced pear (3g fiber)

50-Calorie Portions (cont.)

⅔ cup orange segments (3g fiber)

⅔ cup chopped pineapple (1.5g fiber)

⅔ cup grapefruit sections; about ½ grapefruit (1.5g fiber)

½ cup blueberries (2g fiber)

½ cup cherries (1.5g fiber)

½ cup chopped mango (1.5g fiber)

½ cup grapes; about 15 grapes (0.5g fiber)

⅓ cup sliced banana (1.5g fiber)

⅓ cup pomegranate arils (2.5g fiber)

1½ clementines or other small mandarin oranges (2g fiber)

1 tangerine or other medium mandarin oranges (1.5g fiber)

100-Calorie Portions

2¼ cups chopped watermelon (1.5g fiber)

2 cups halved strawberries; about 17 large strawberries (6g fiber)

1¾ cups sliced apple; about 1 medium apple (4.5g fiber)

1¾ cups chopped cantaloupe (2.5g fiber)

1⅔ cups blackberries (12.5g fiber)

100-Calorie Portions (cont.)

1⅔ cups sliced peaches; about 2 small peaches (4g fiber)

1⅔ cups chopped honeydew melon (2g fiber)

1½ cups raspberries (12g fiber)

1½ cups sliced nectarines; about 1½ medium nectarines (3.5g fiber)

1¼ cups sliced pear; about 1 medium pear (5.5g fiber)

1¼ cups orange segments; 1½ medium oranges (5.5g fiber)

1¼ cups blueberries (4.5g fiber)

1¼ cups chopped pineapple (3g fiber)

1 cup grapefruit sections; about 1 grapefruit (3.5g fiber)

1 cup cherries (3g fiber)

1 cup chopped mango; about ½ mango (2.5g fiber)

1 cup grapes; about 30 grapes (1.5g fiber)

¾ cup sliced banana; about 1 medium banana (3g fiber)

⅔ cup pomegranate arils; about ½ pomegranate (4.5g fiber)

Look for 100-calorie containers of POM POMs, ready-to-eat arils!

3 clementines or other small mandarin oranges (3.5g fiber)

2 tangerines or other medium mandarin oranges (3.5g fiber)

Pssst... Fruits with high fiber counts and large serving sizes tend to be the most filling.

HG's Veggie Charts

Select your favorites when recipes call for your choice from these charts! And remember to scope out the Seasonal Produce Guide on page 313 . . .

High-Fiber Veggies

Tomatoes

Onions

Bell peppers

Green beans

Sugar snap peas

Snow peas

Bean sprouts

Broccoli

Brussels sprouts

Carrots

Jicama

High-Volume Veggies

Mushrooms

Cucumbers

Cabbage

Celery

Zucchini

Eggplant

Yellow squash

Asparagus

Cauliflower

Kale

Spinach

THAT'S ALL FOR NOW!

There you have it . . . a whopping 200 new recipes
for the Hungry Girl Diet! Try 'em all, and let me know which ones
you love the most! If you have questions, comments,
or just want to say hi, email me at **ask@hungry-girl.com**.
For up-to-the-minute recipes, food finds, tips 'n tricks, and more,
sign up for free daily emails at **hungry-girl.com**!

'Til next time . . . Chew the right thing!

Lisa :)

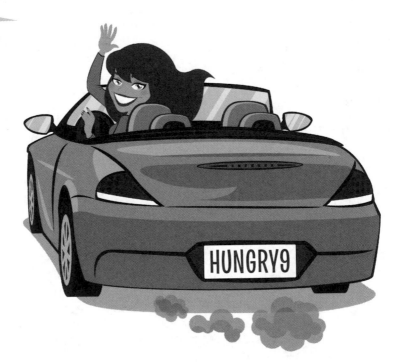

Index